PICTURE BOOK OF
Baking Goodies

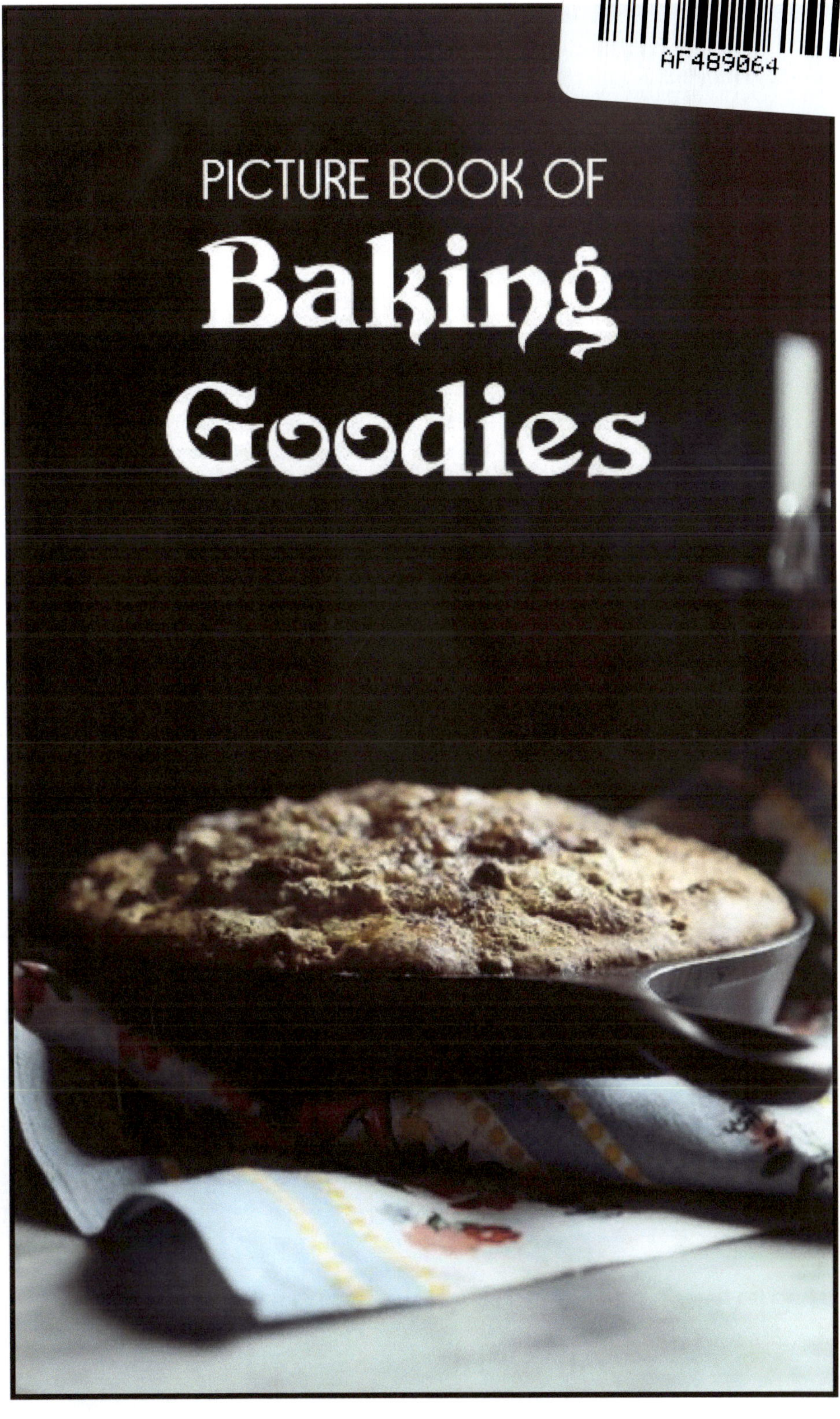

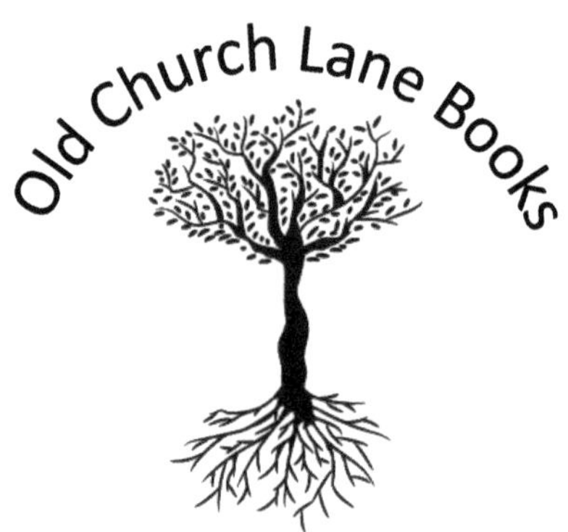
Old Church Lane Books

Cast Iron Baking

Apple Pie Prep

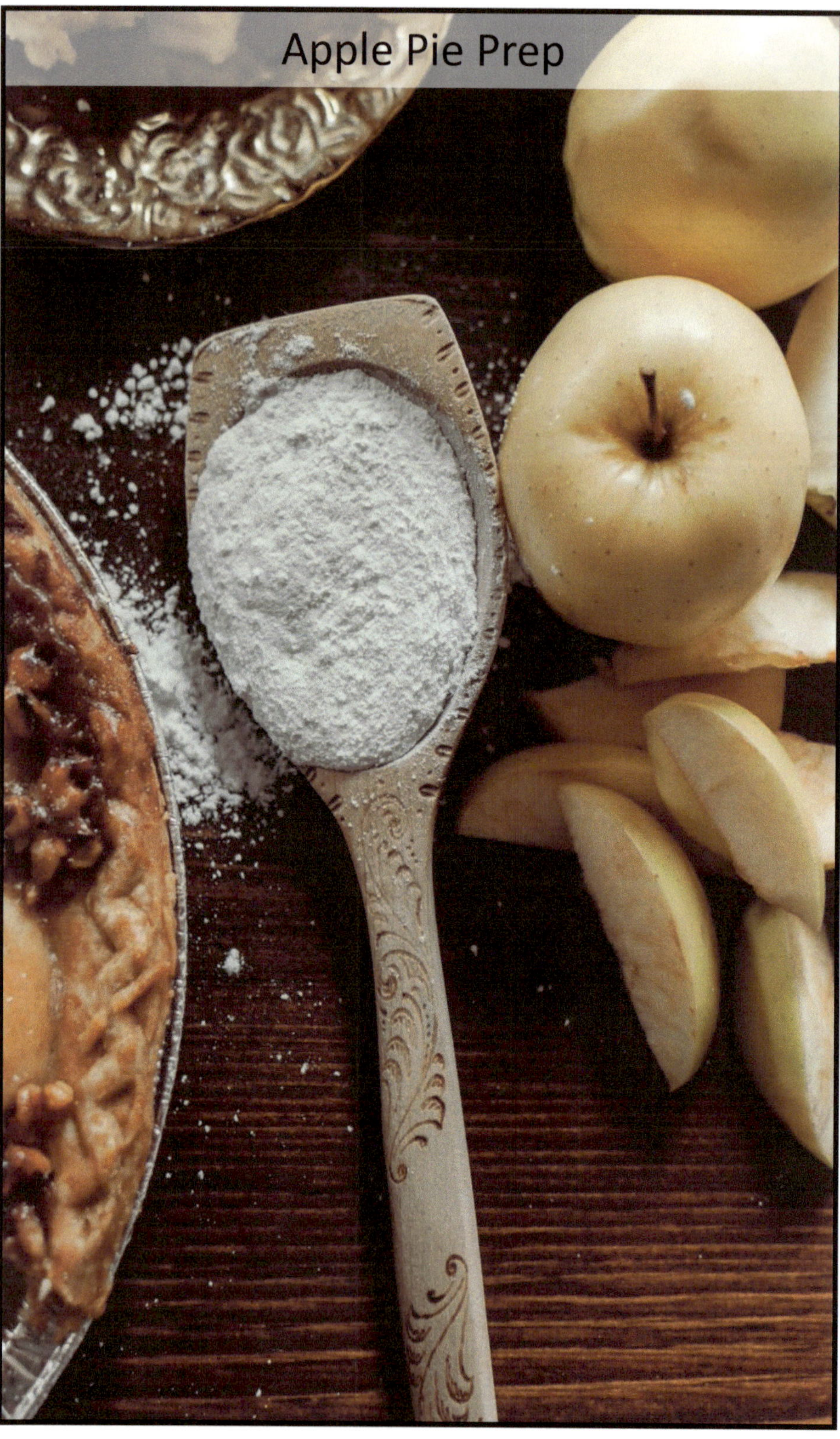

Lemon Squares

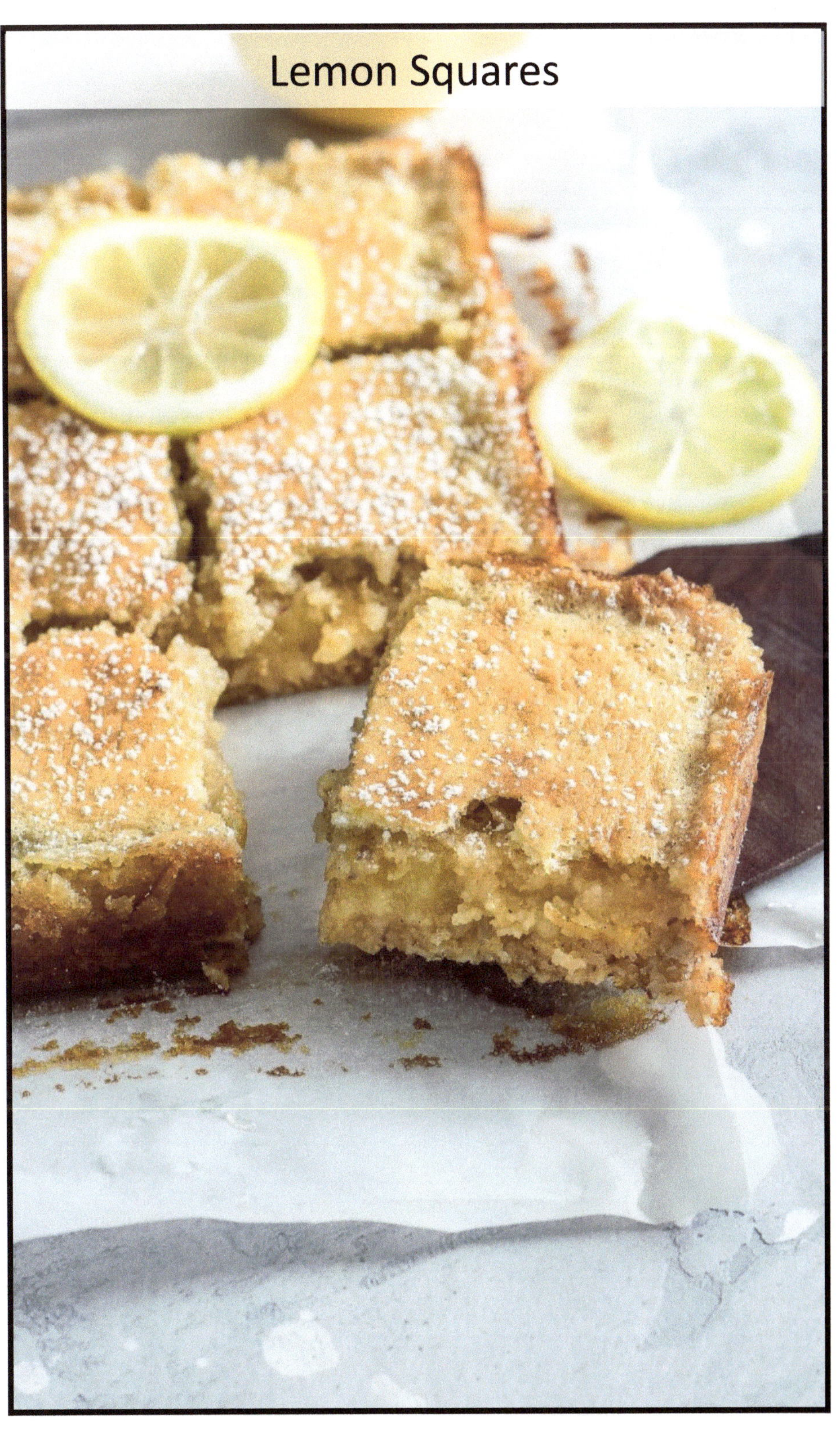

Sifting

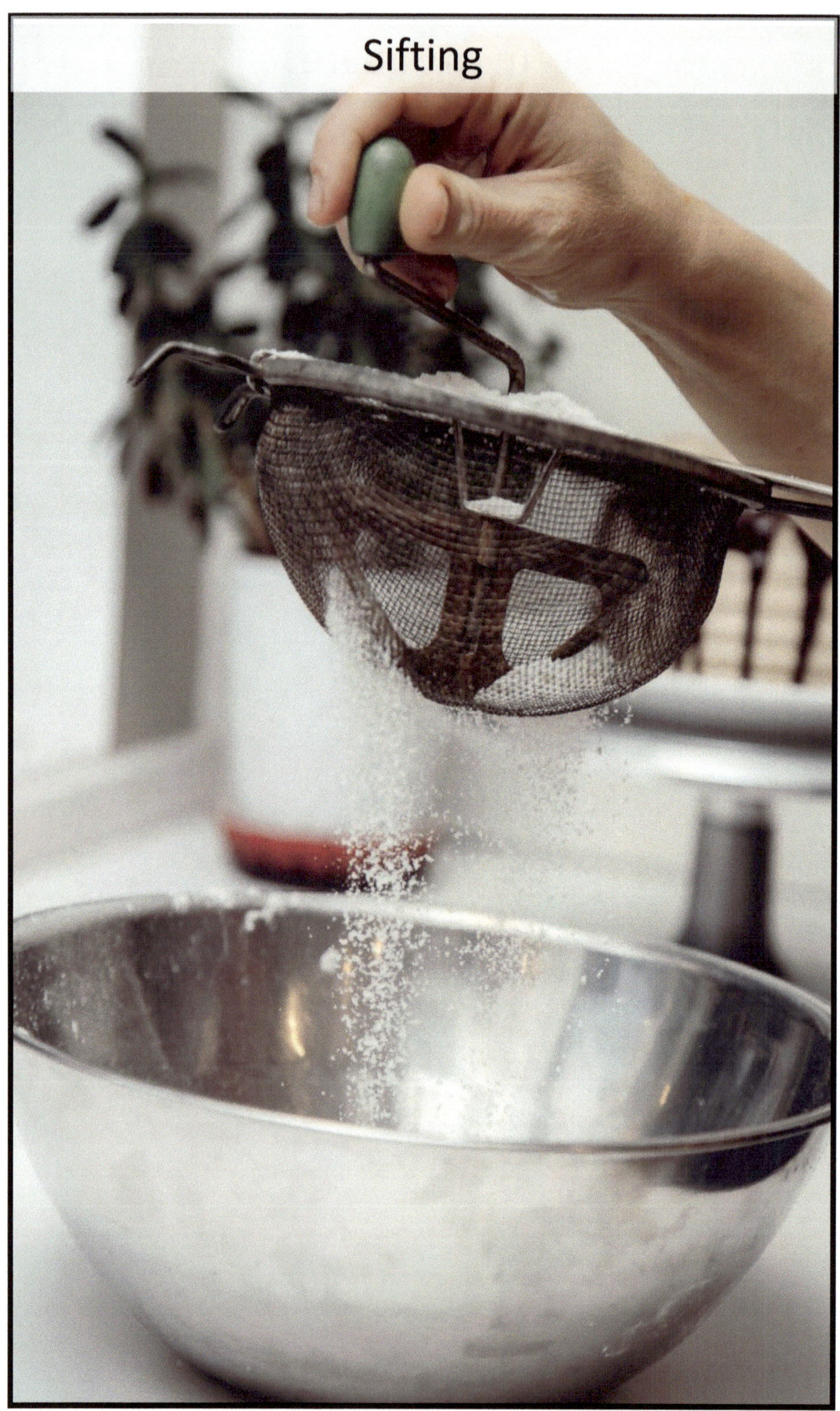

Chocolate Chip Cookies

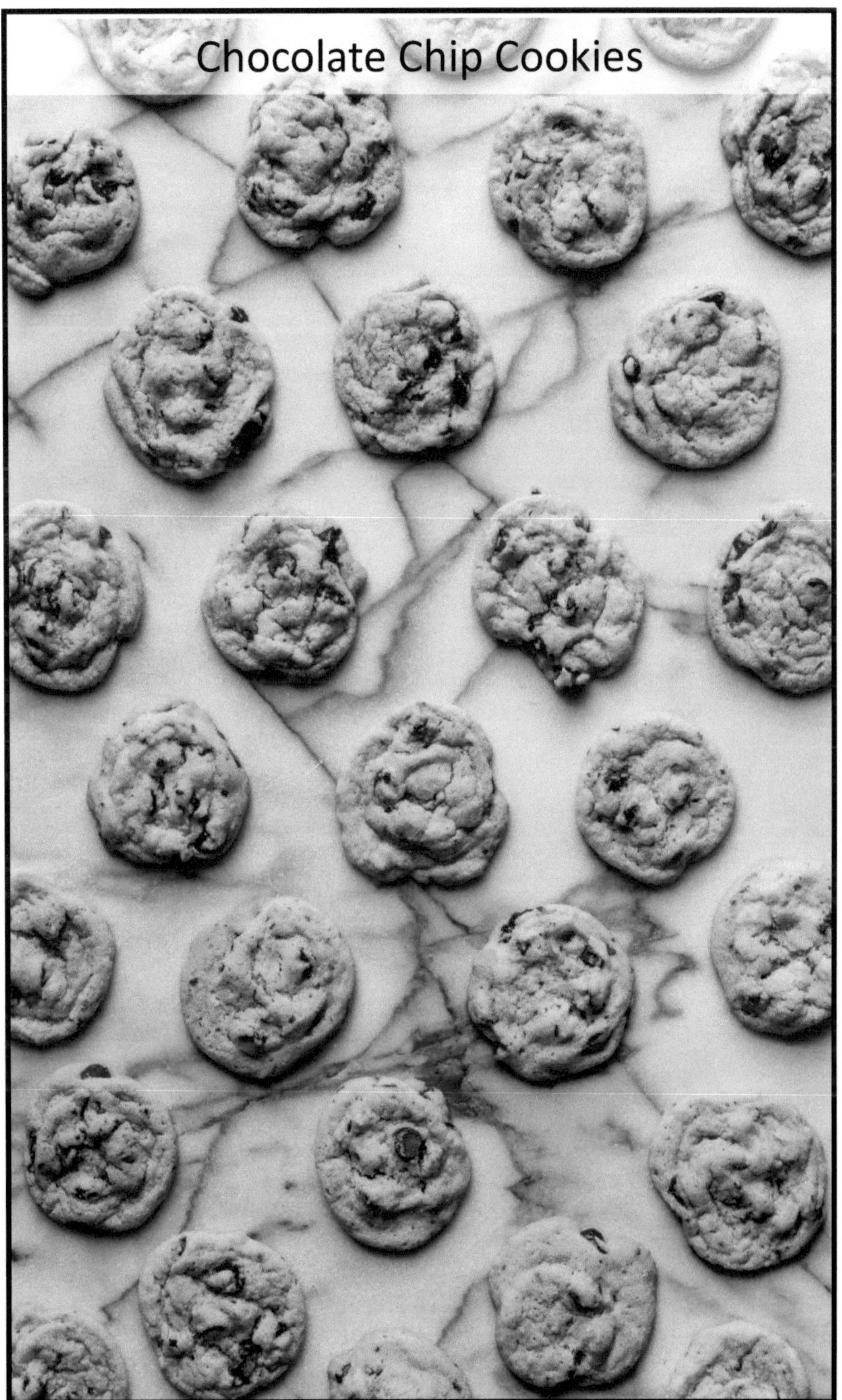

Apple Pie

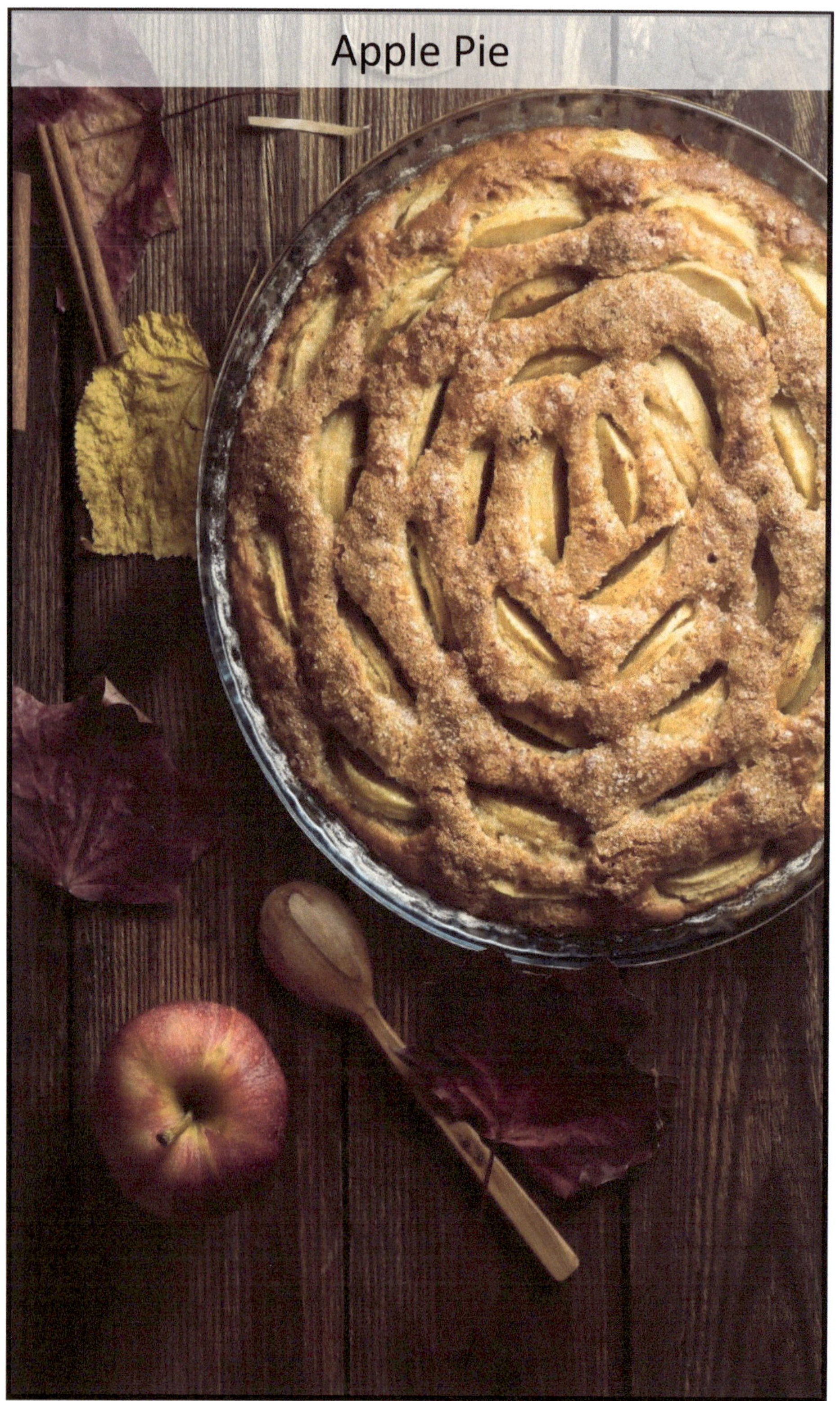

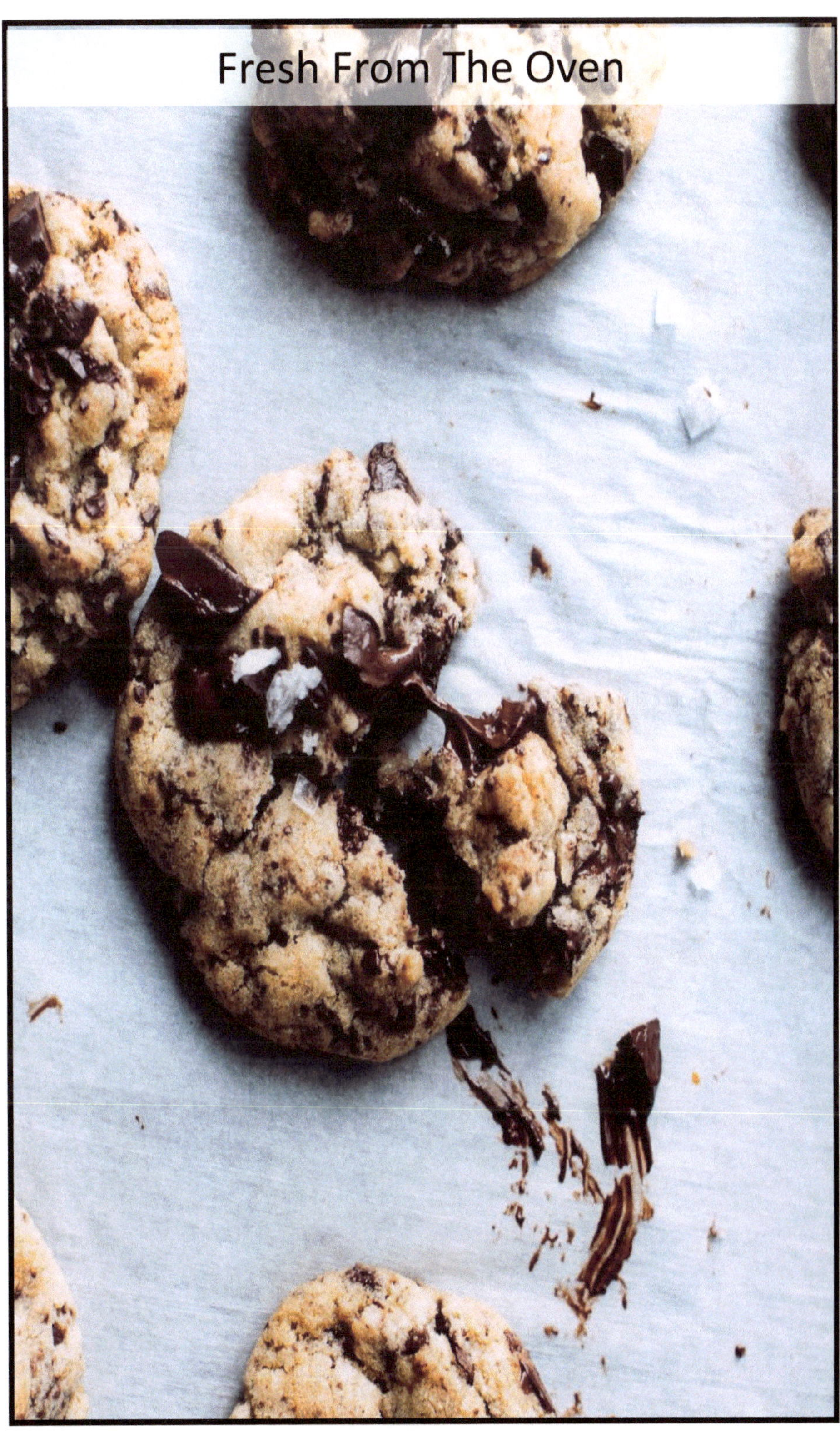

Cookie Cutter

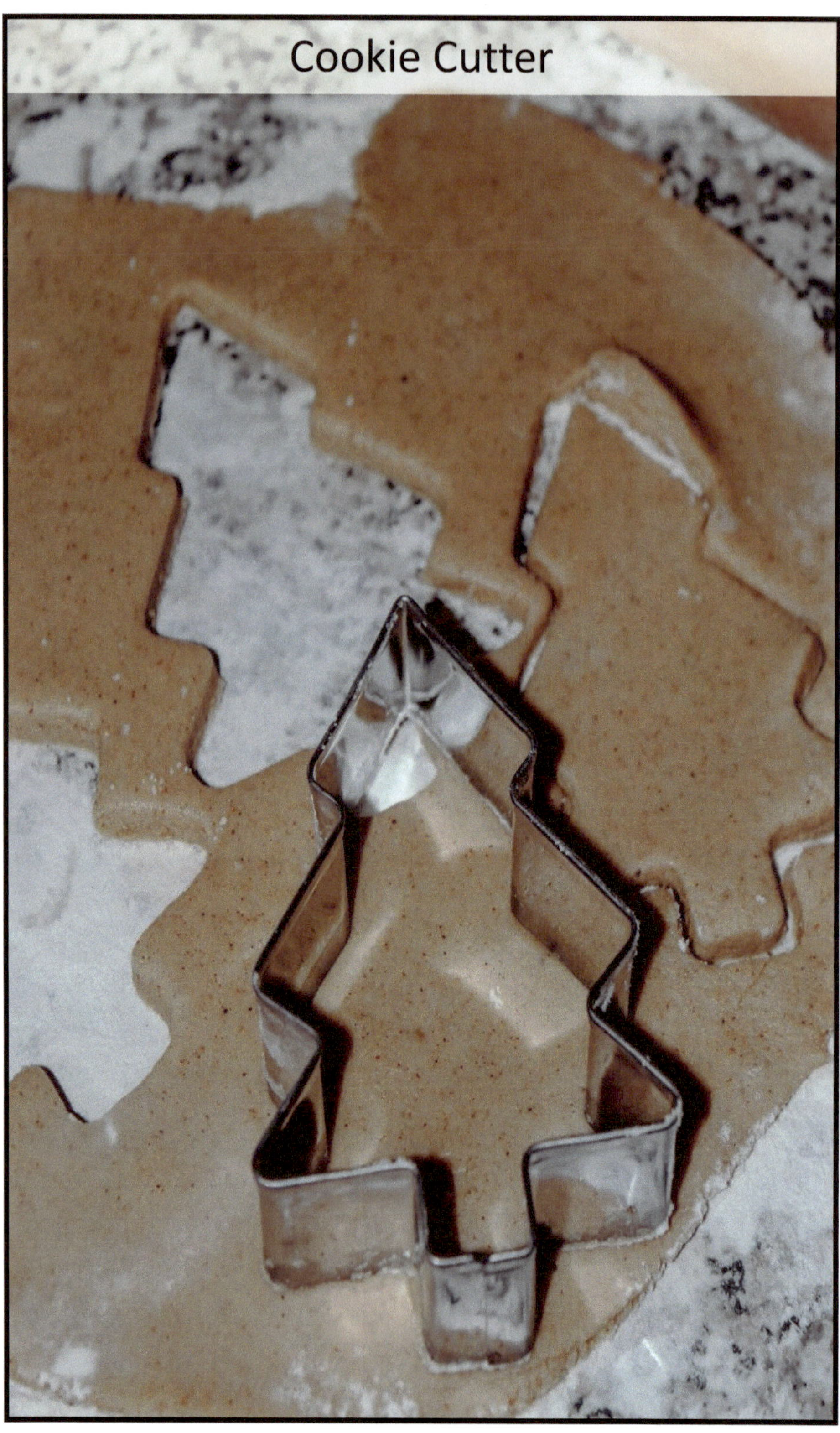

Decorated Cookies

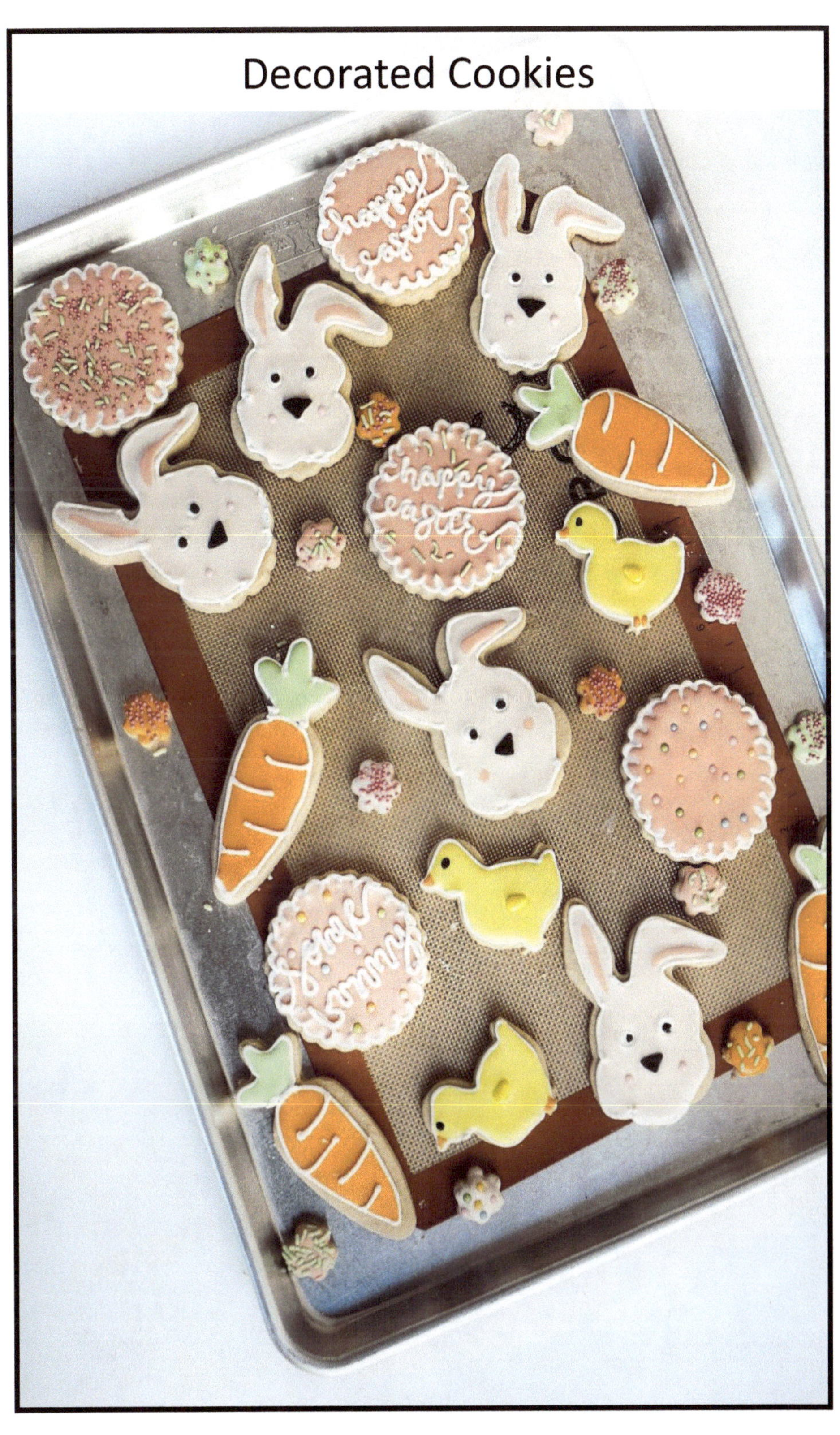

Egg In The Well

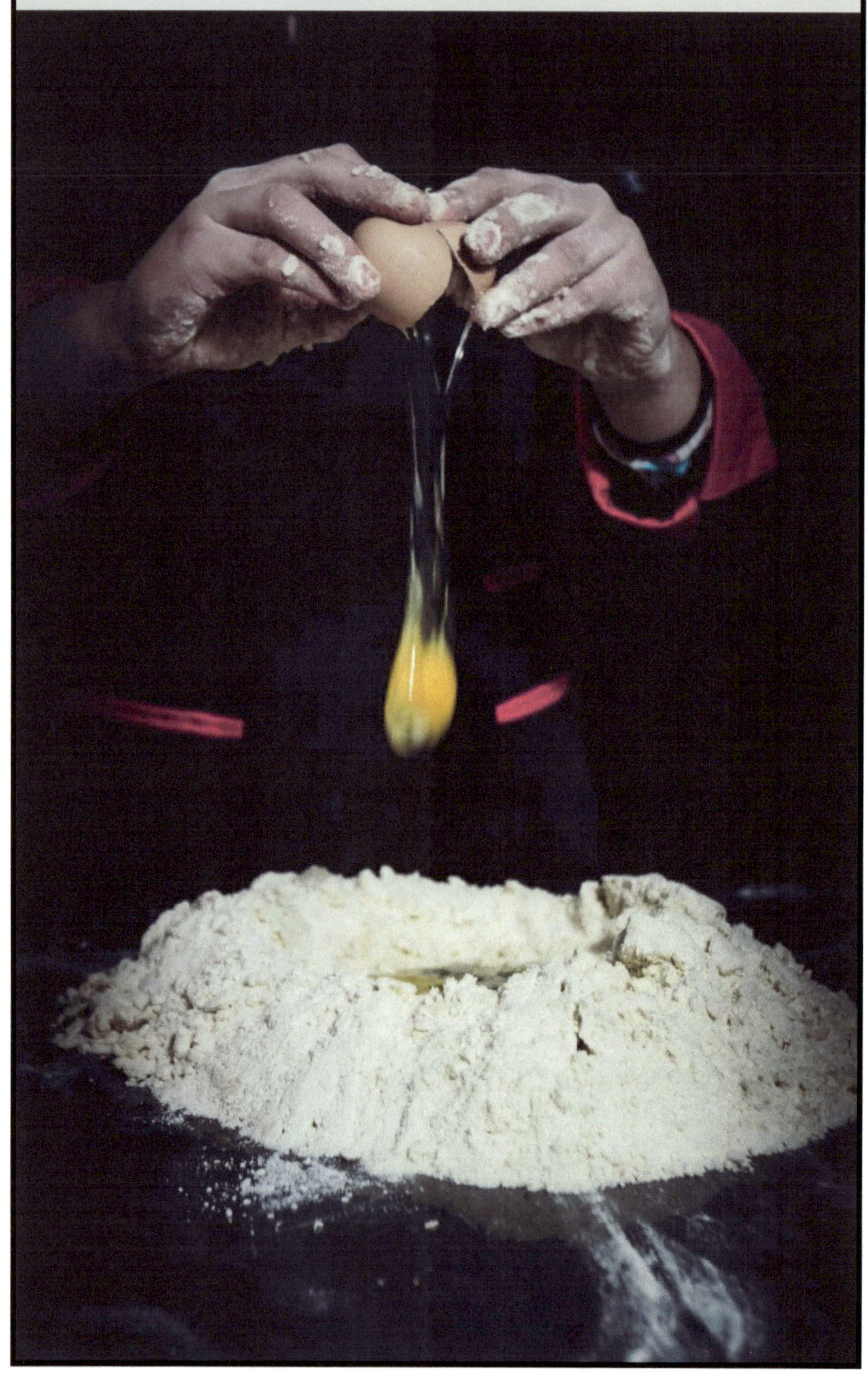

Pumpkin Pie

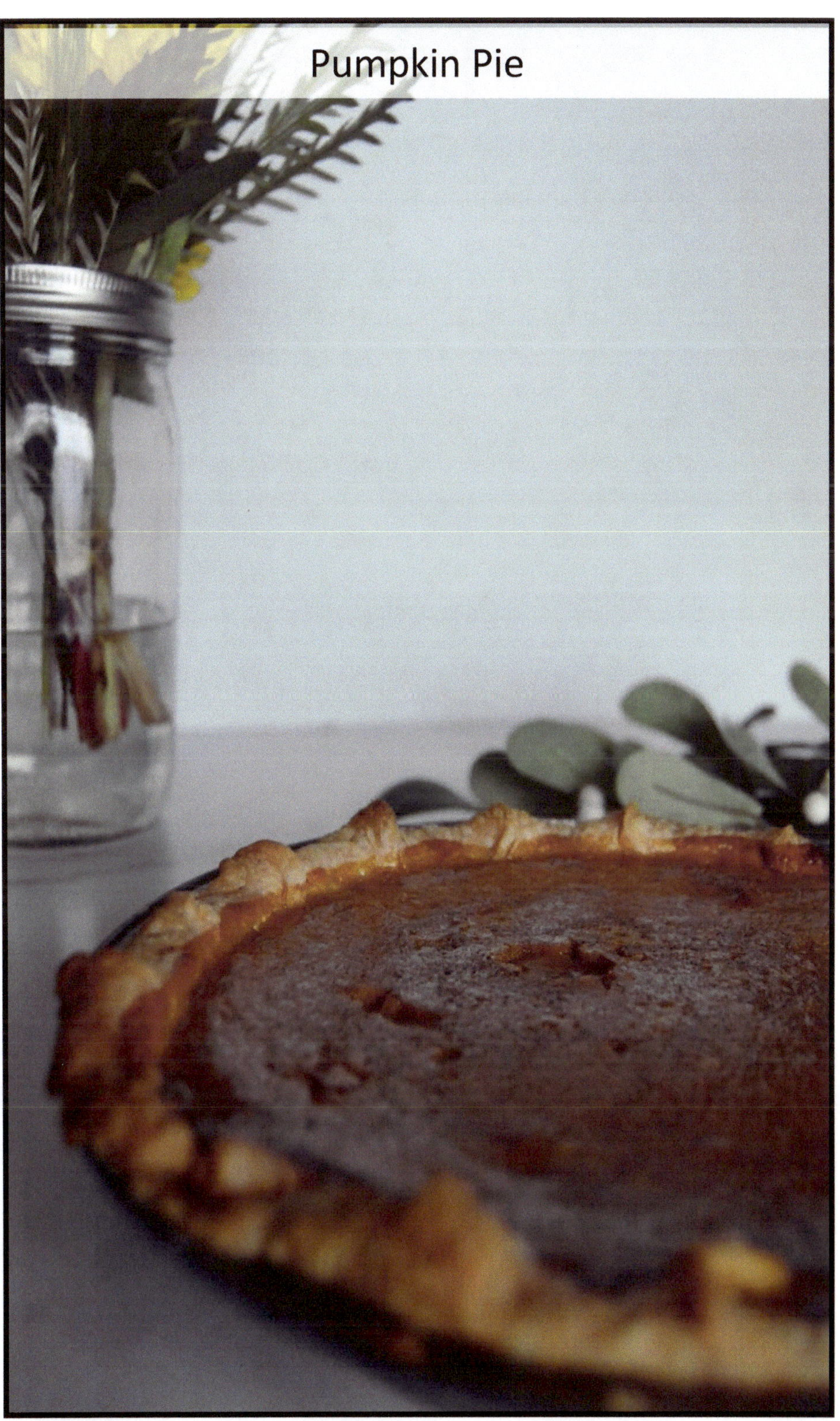

Cinnamon Rolls

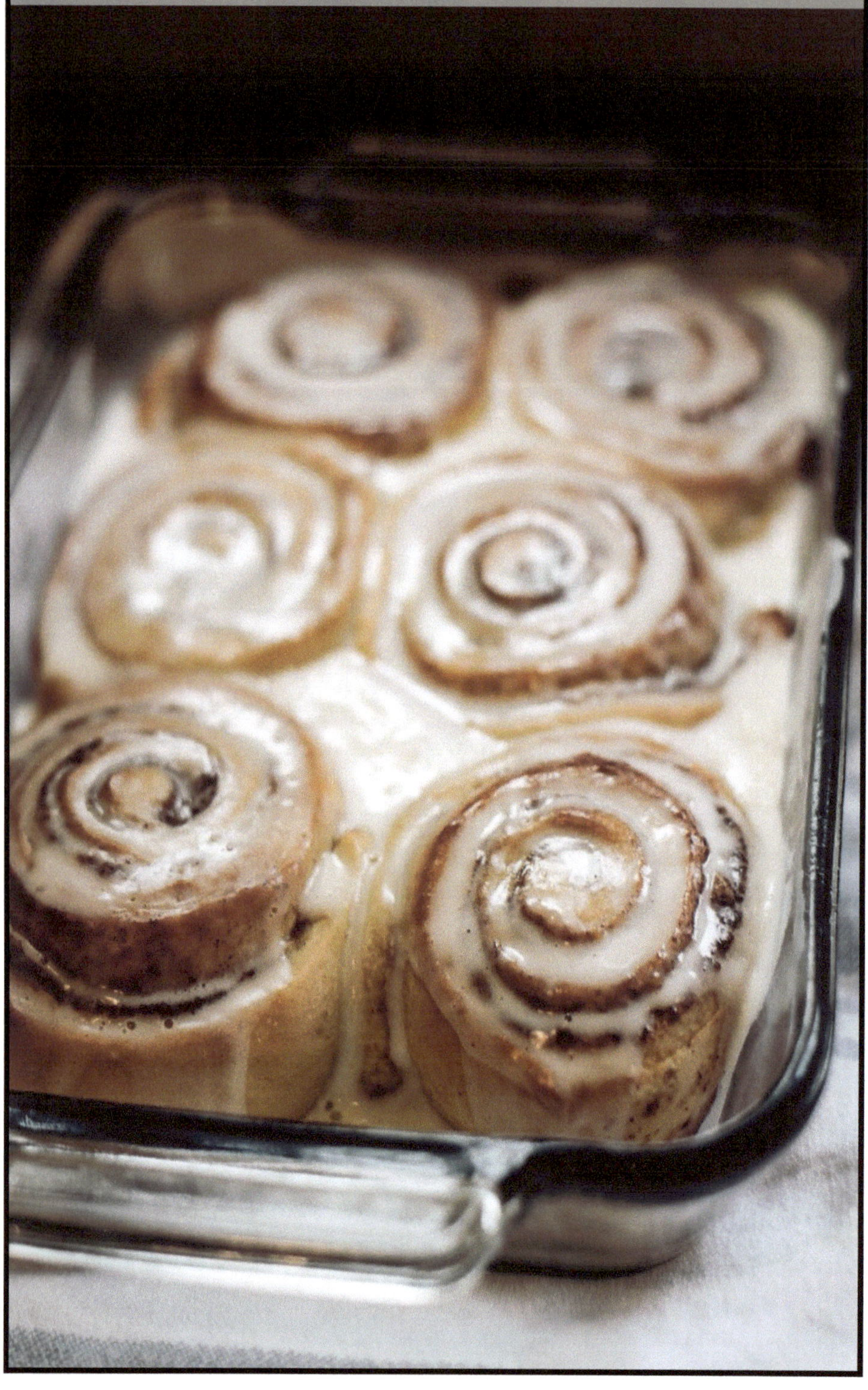

Candy Kiss Cookies

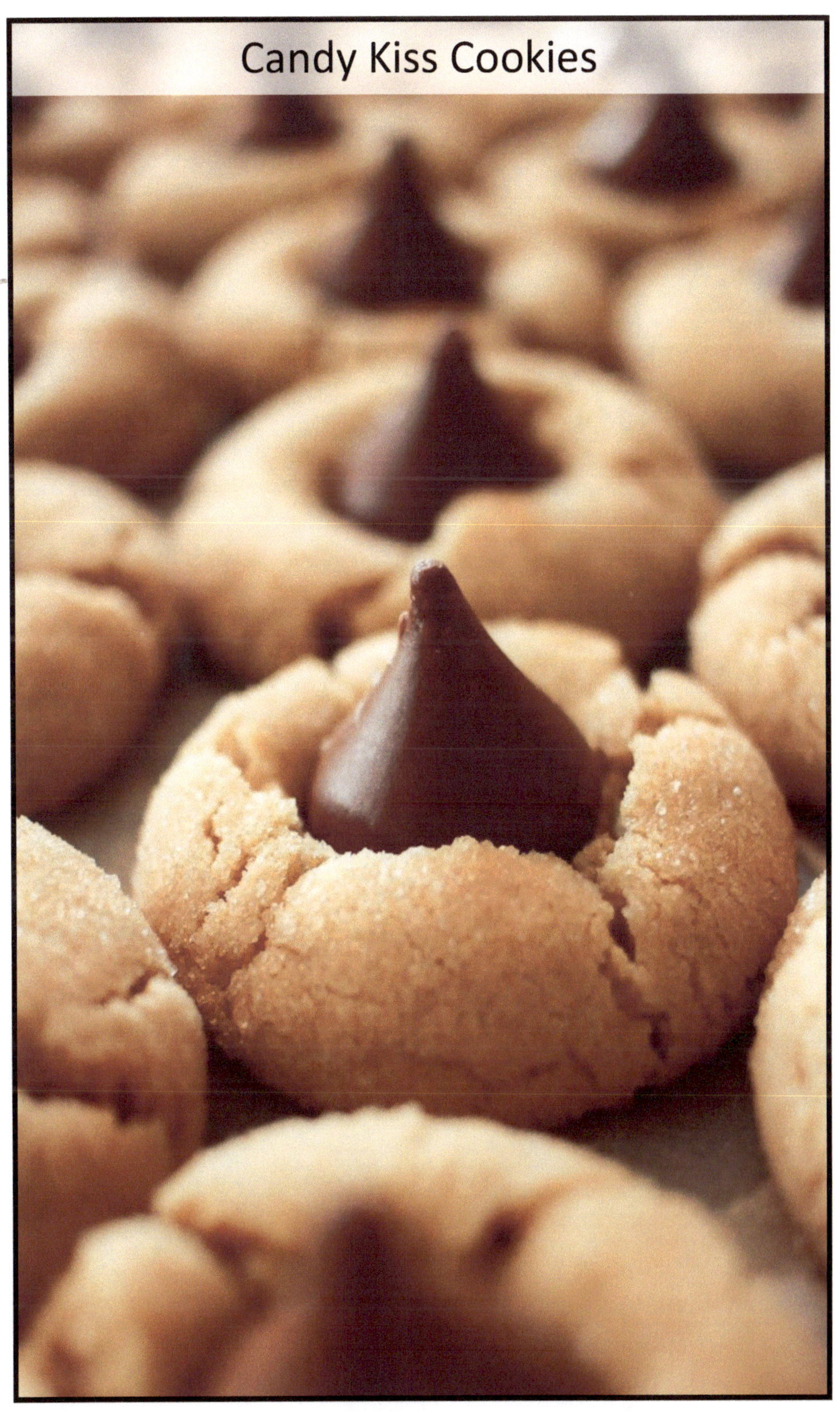

Cookie Tin Gifts

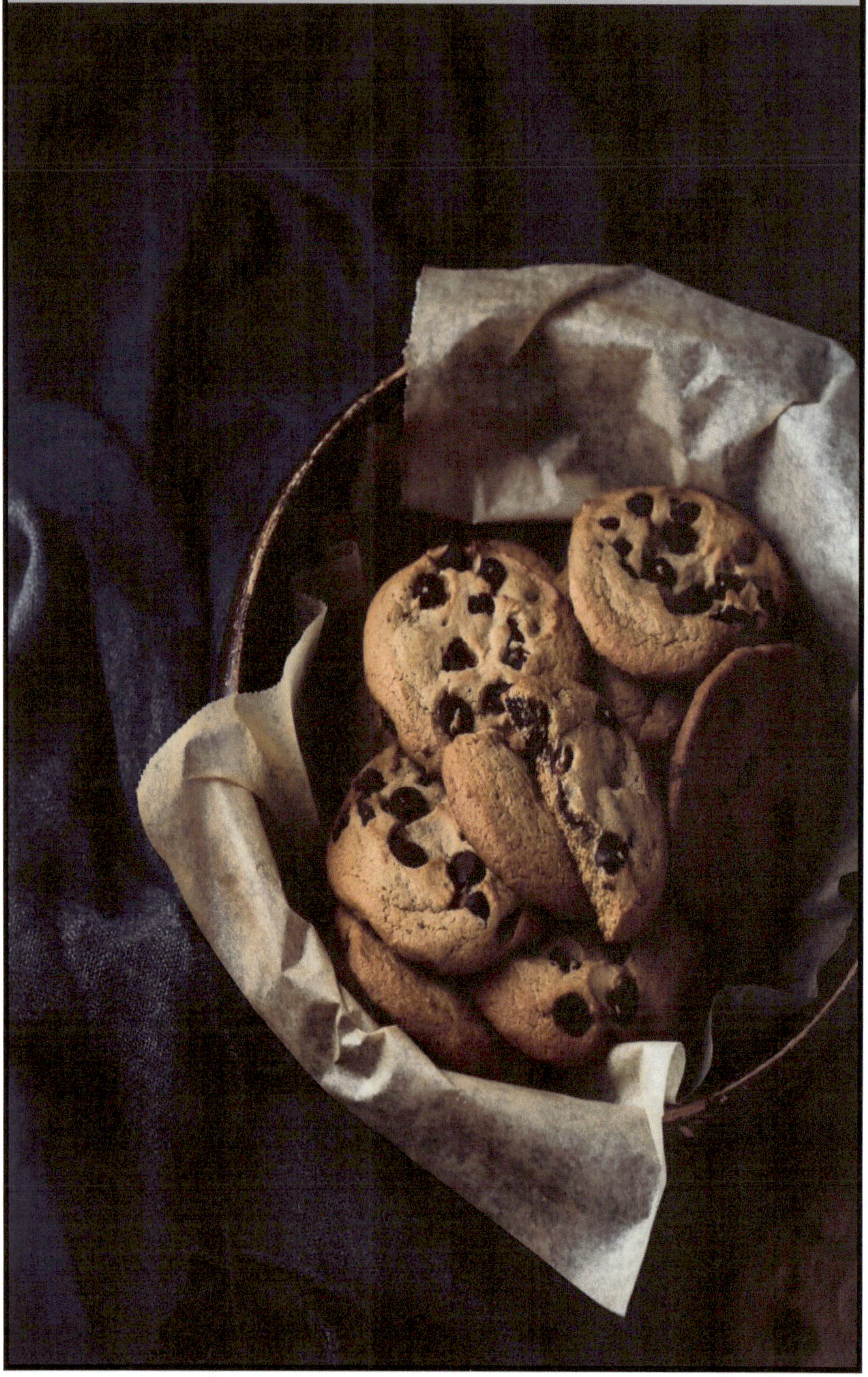

Honey Sweets

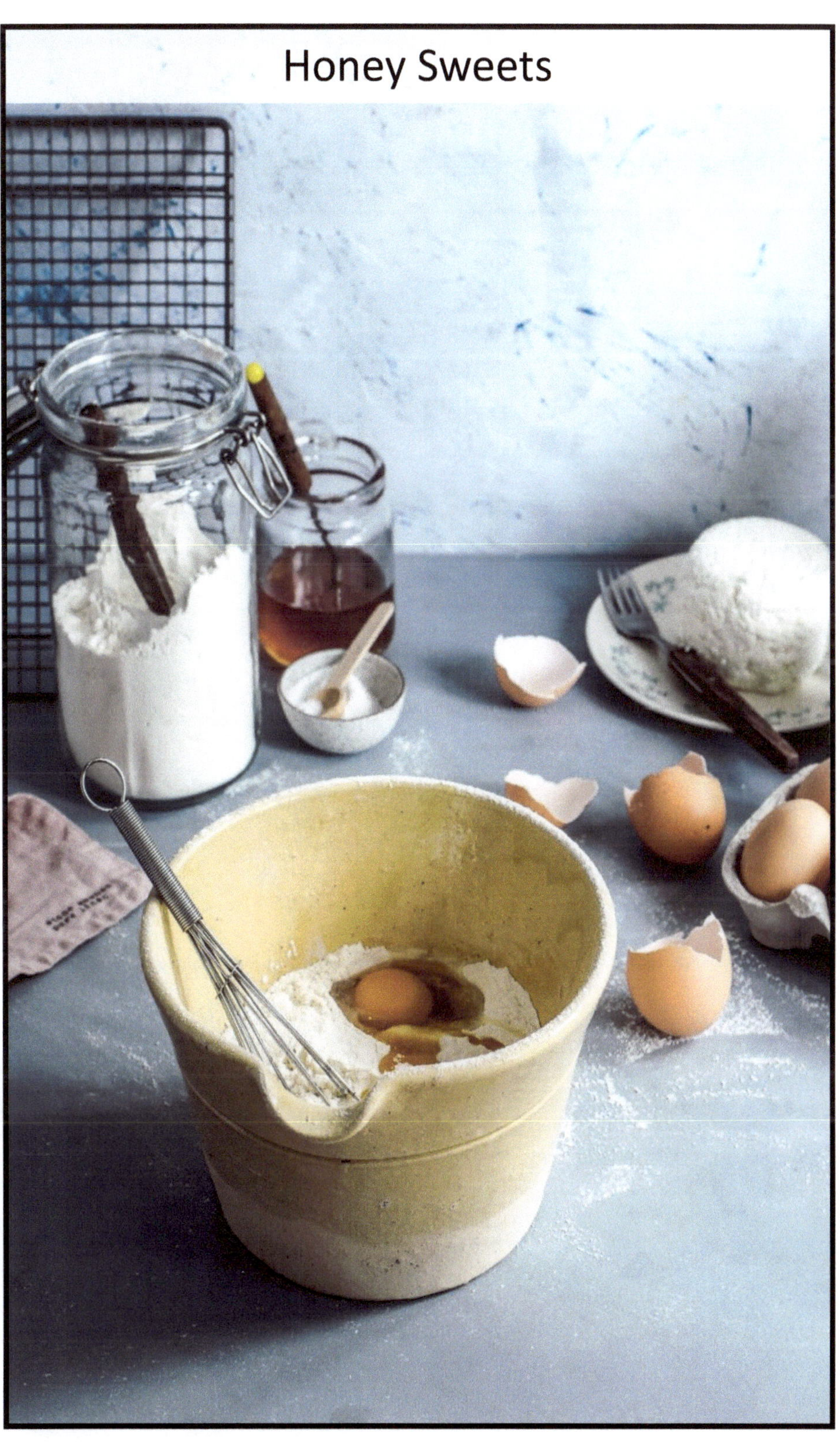

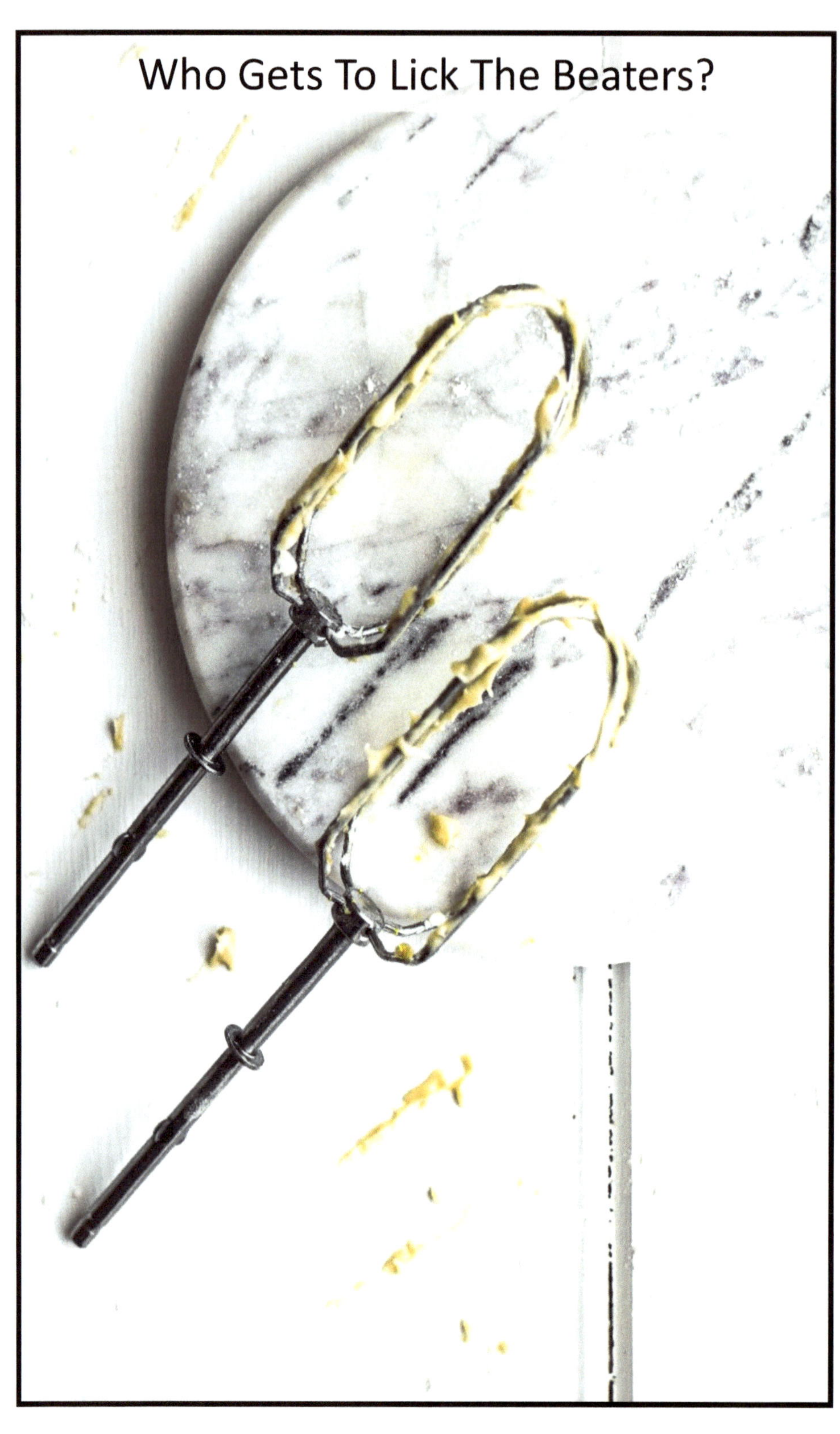

Who Gets To Lick The Beaters?

Rolling Out The Dough

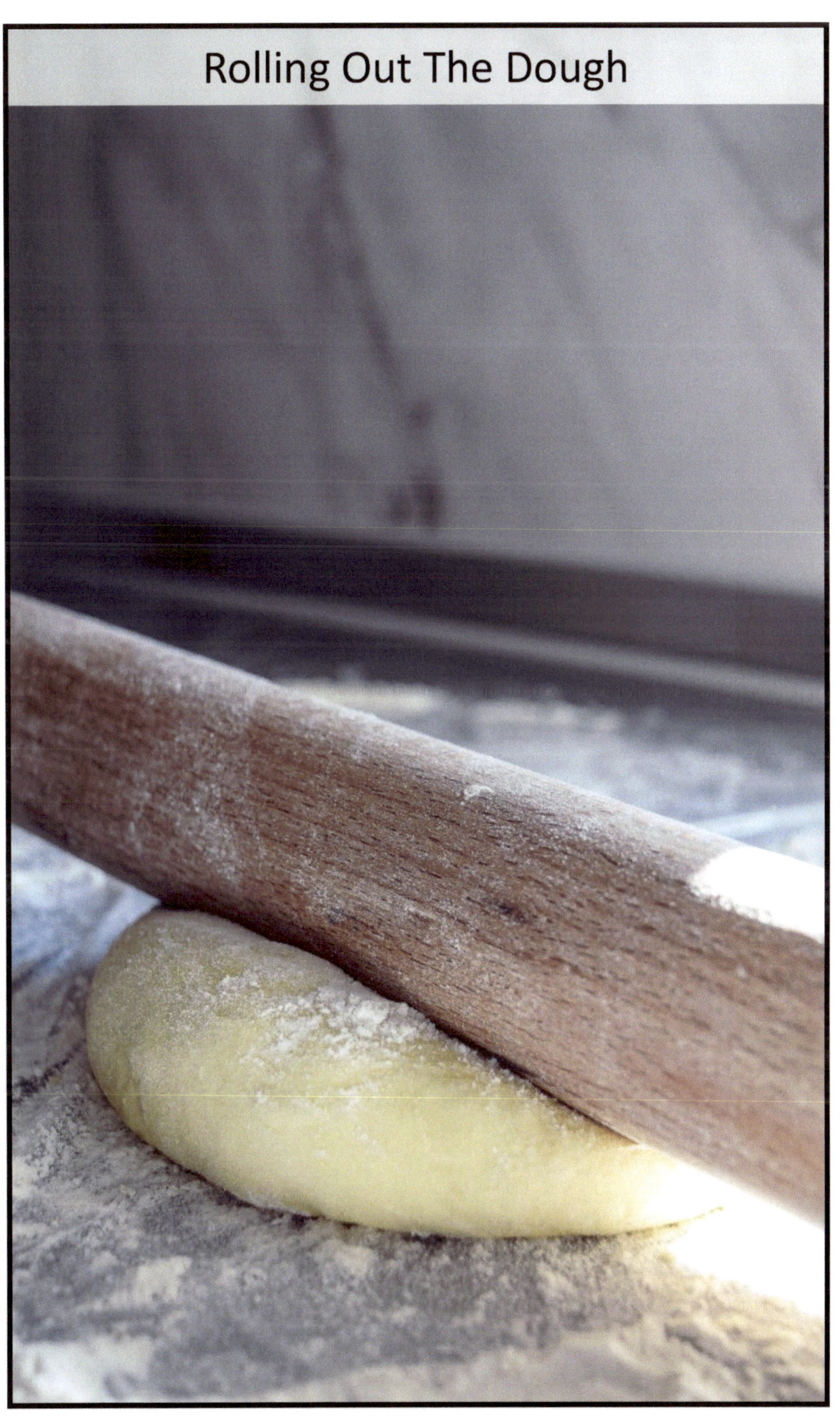

Peanut Butter Cookies

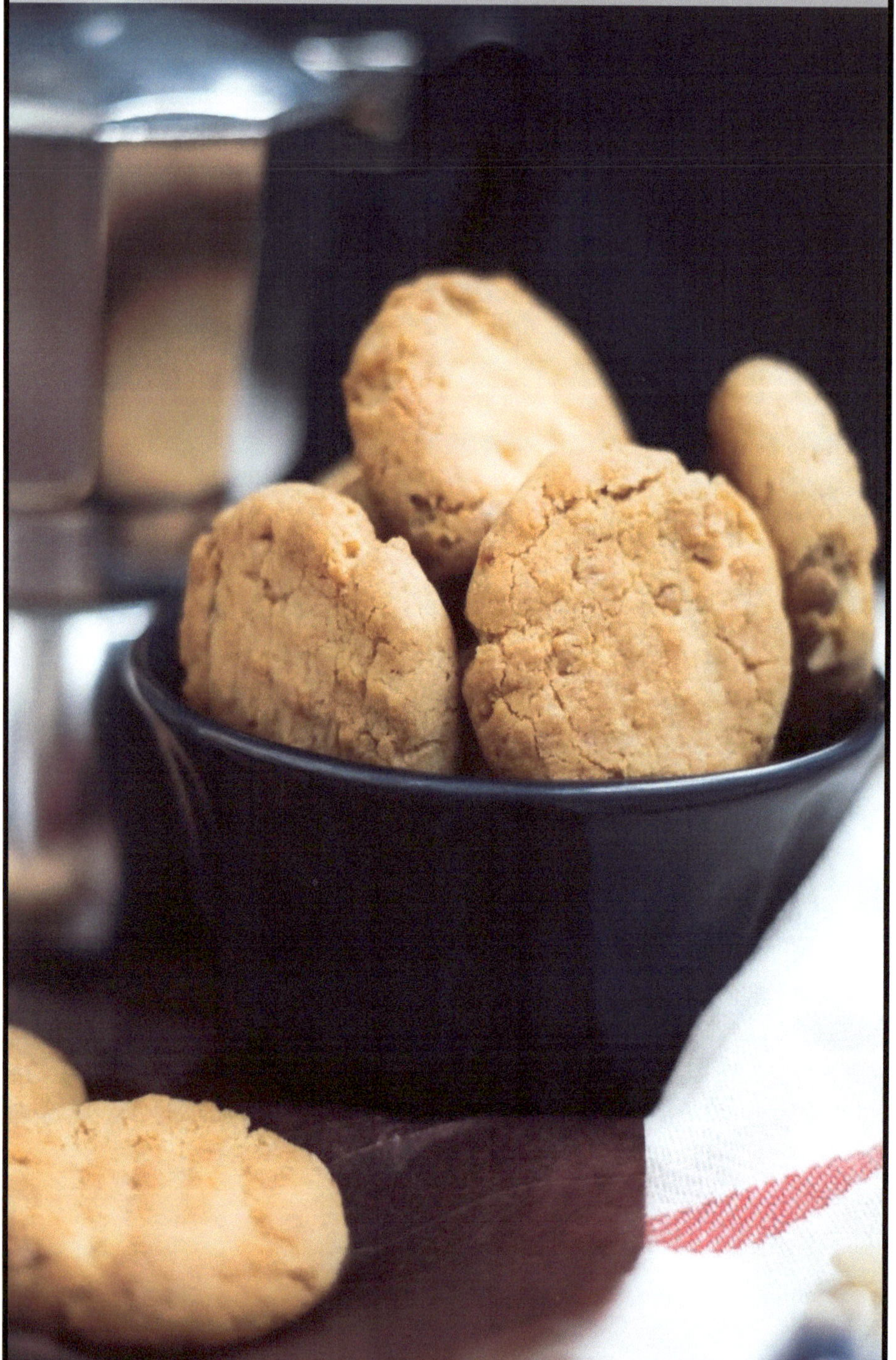

Sweet Loaf Bread

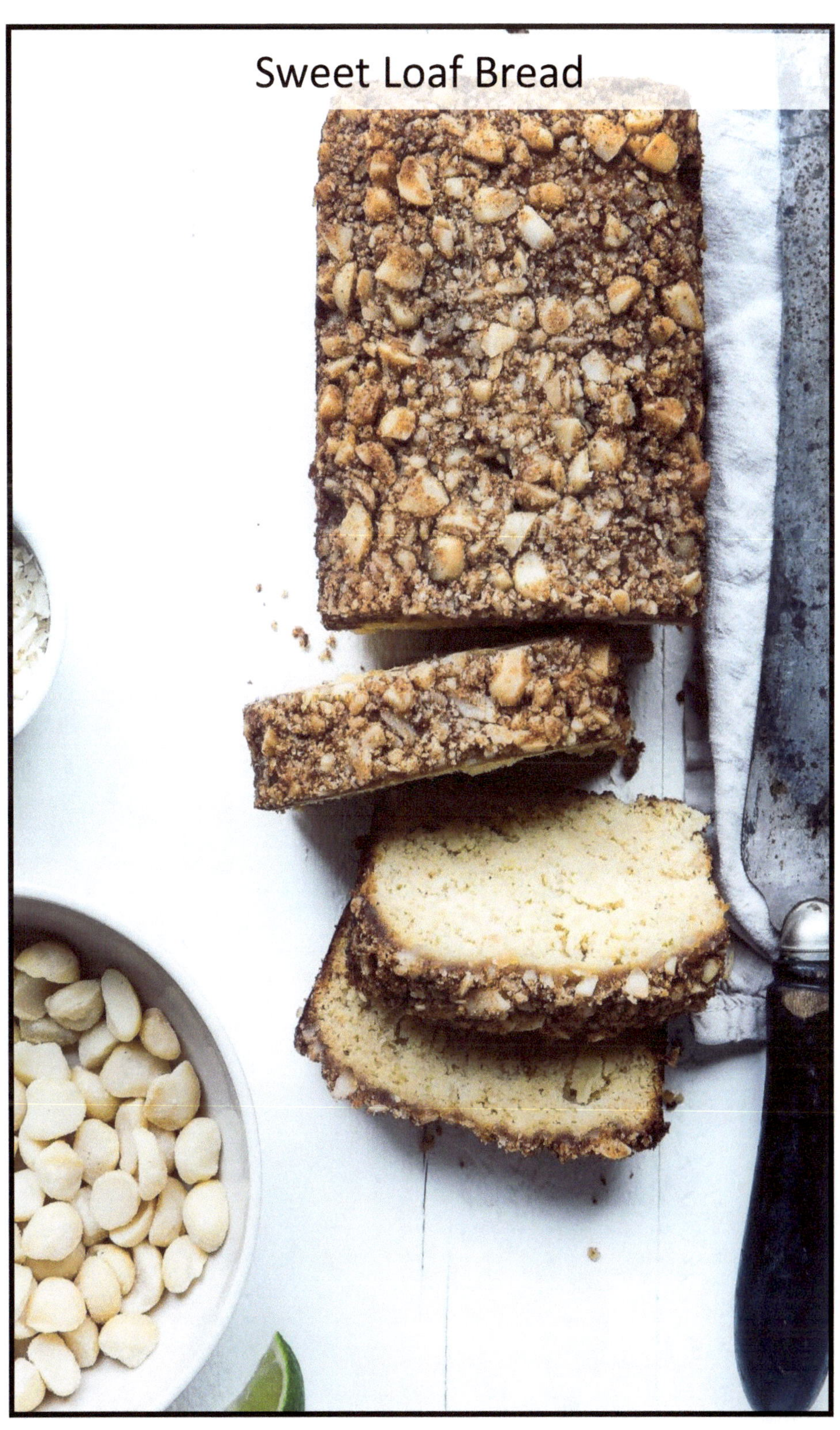

Fresh Bread

Scones

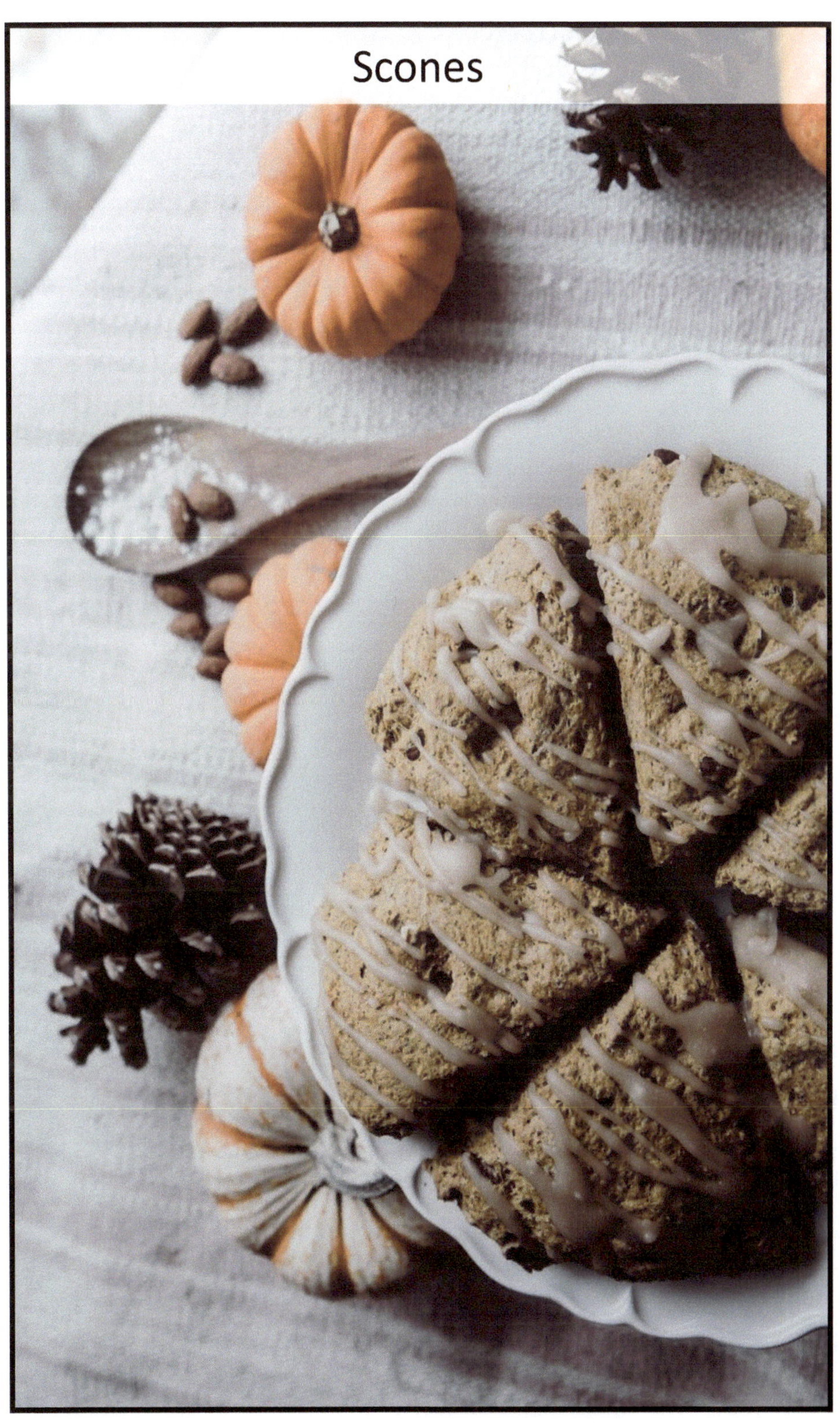

Oatmeal Cookies

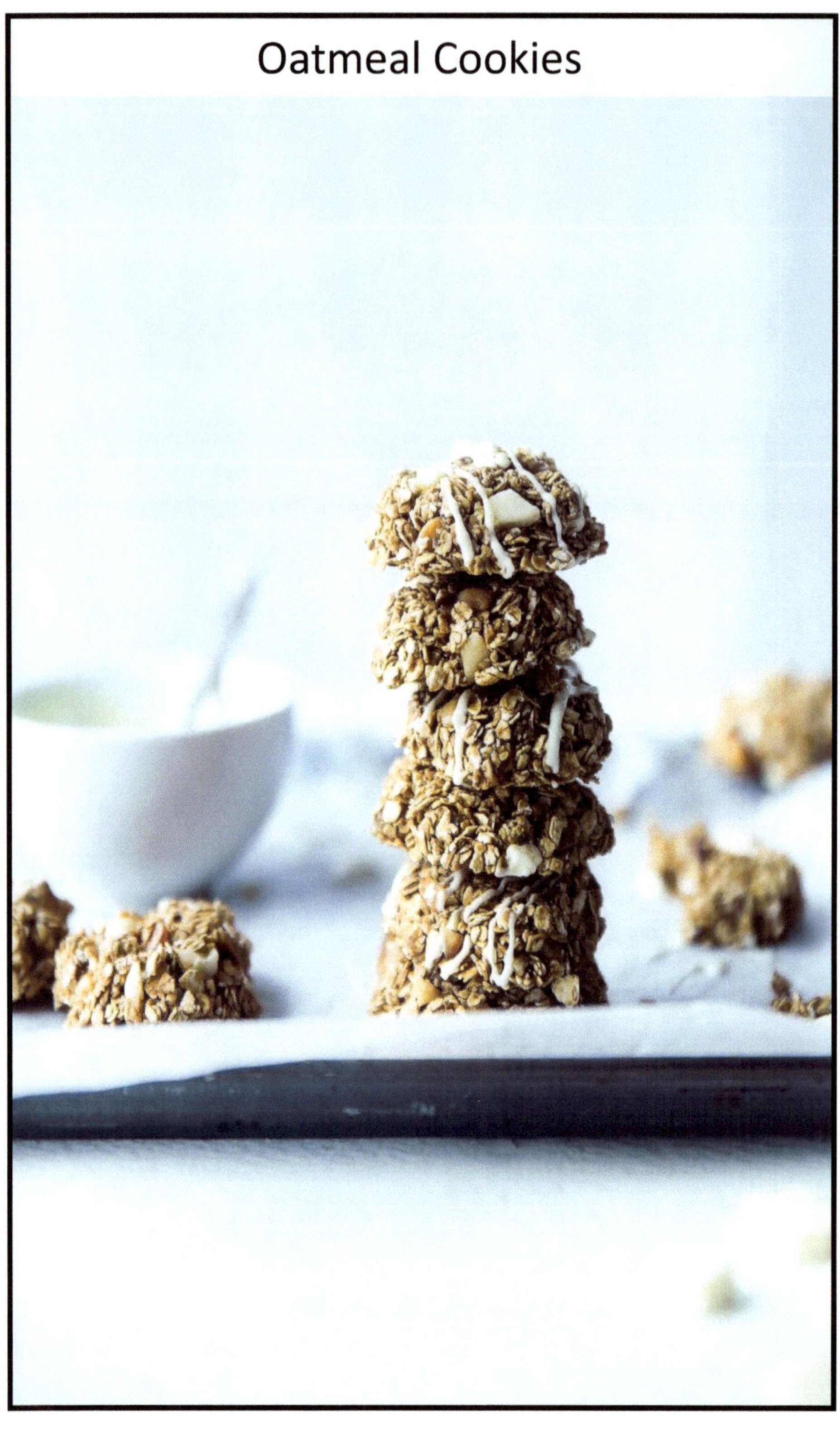

Raspberry Muffins

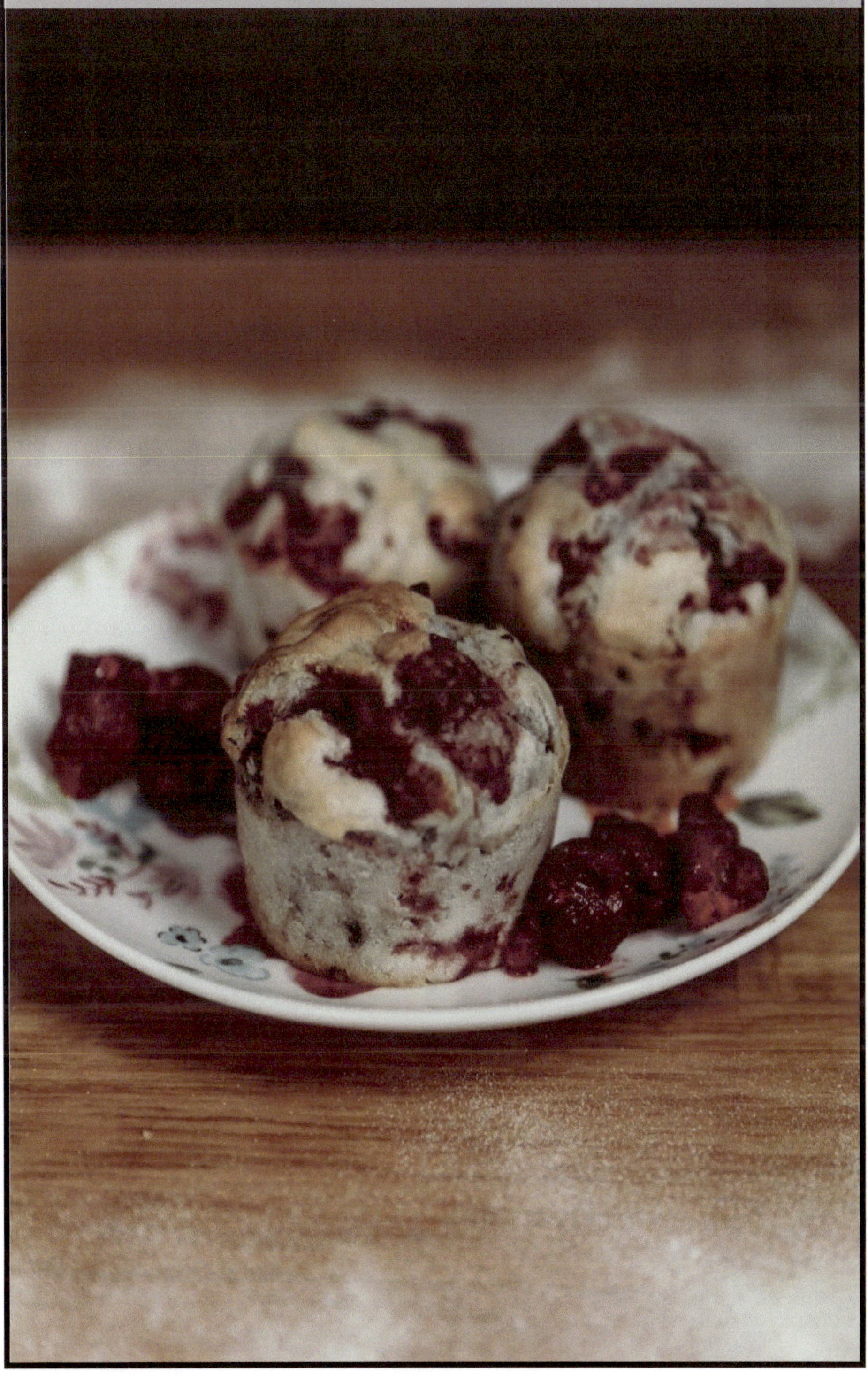

Peanut Butter and Chocolate Cookies

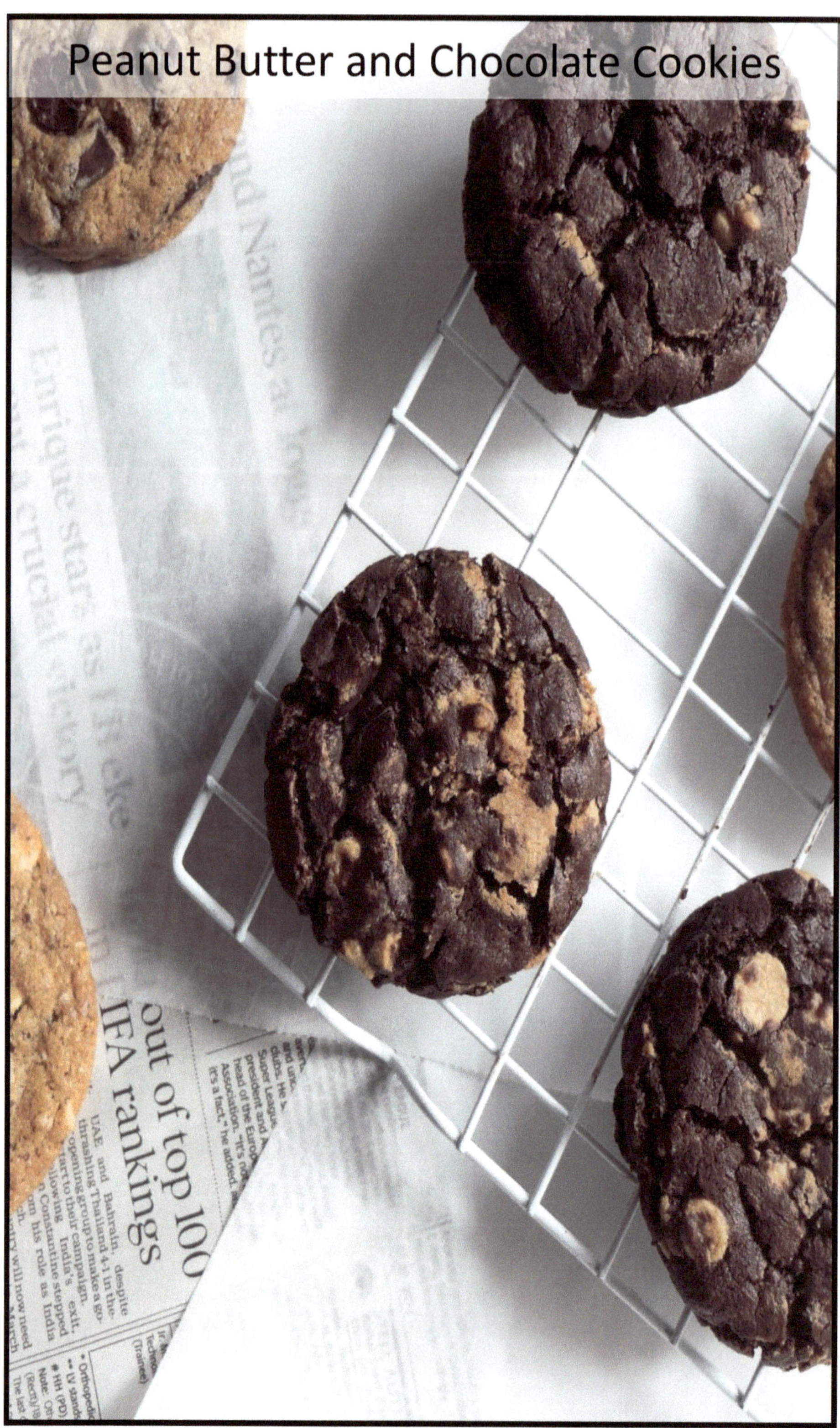

Corn Muffins

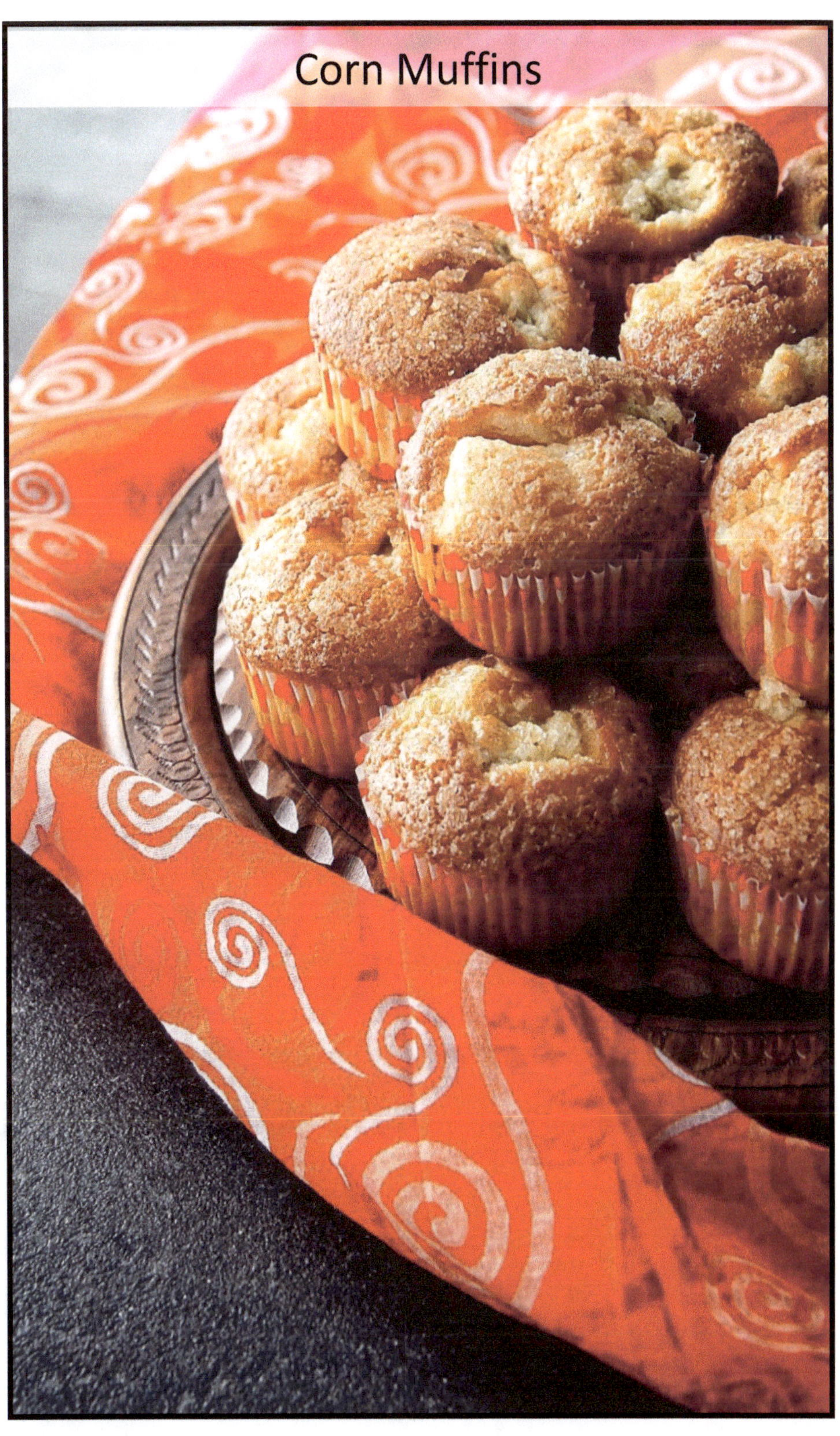

Blueberry Muffins

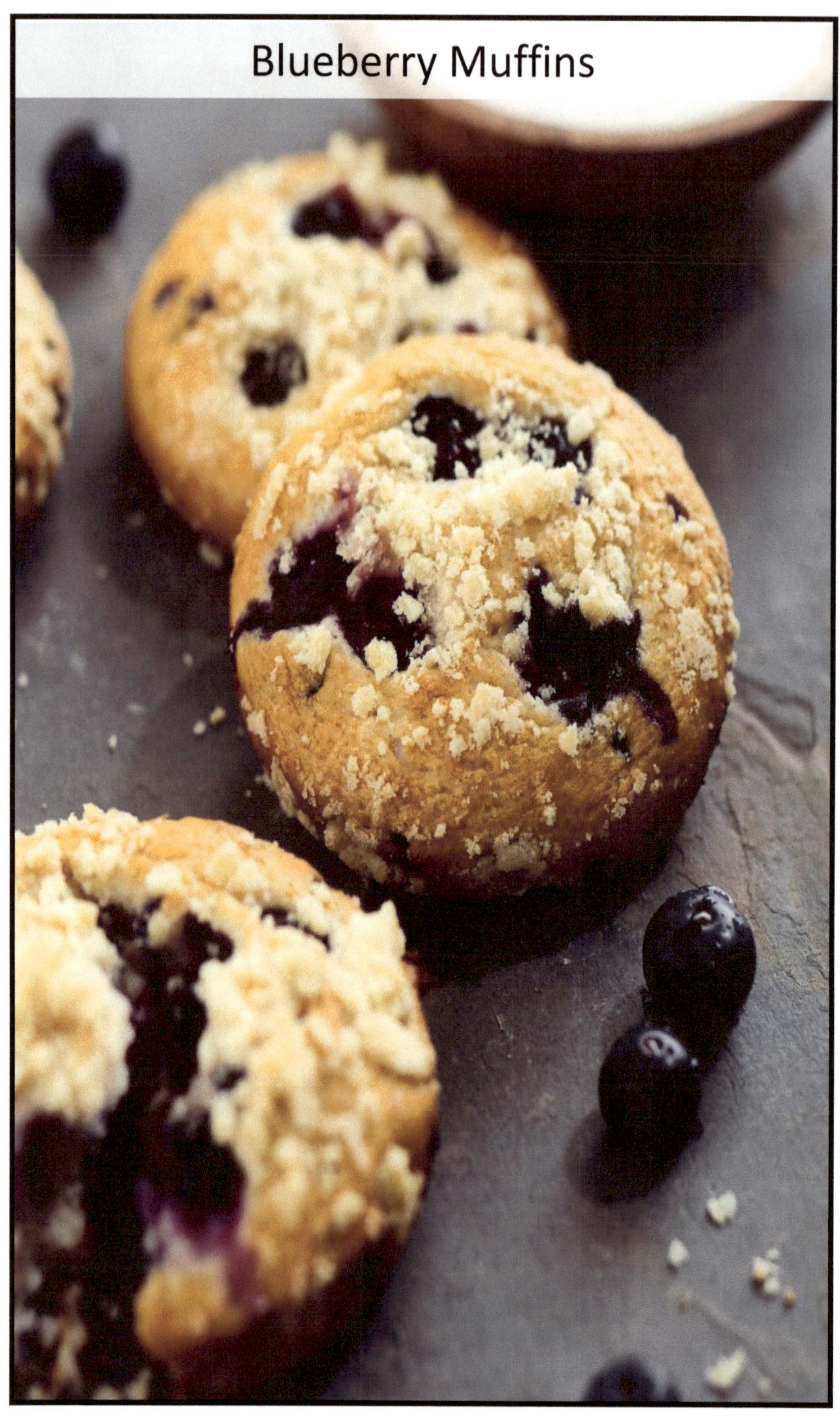

Berry Pie

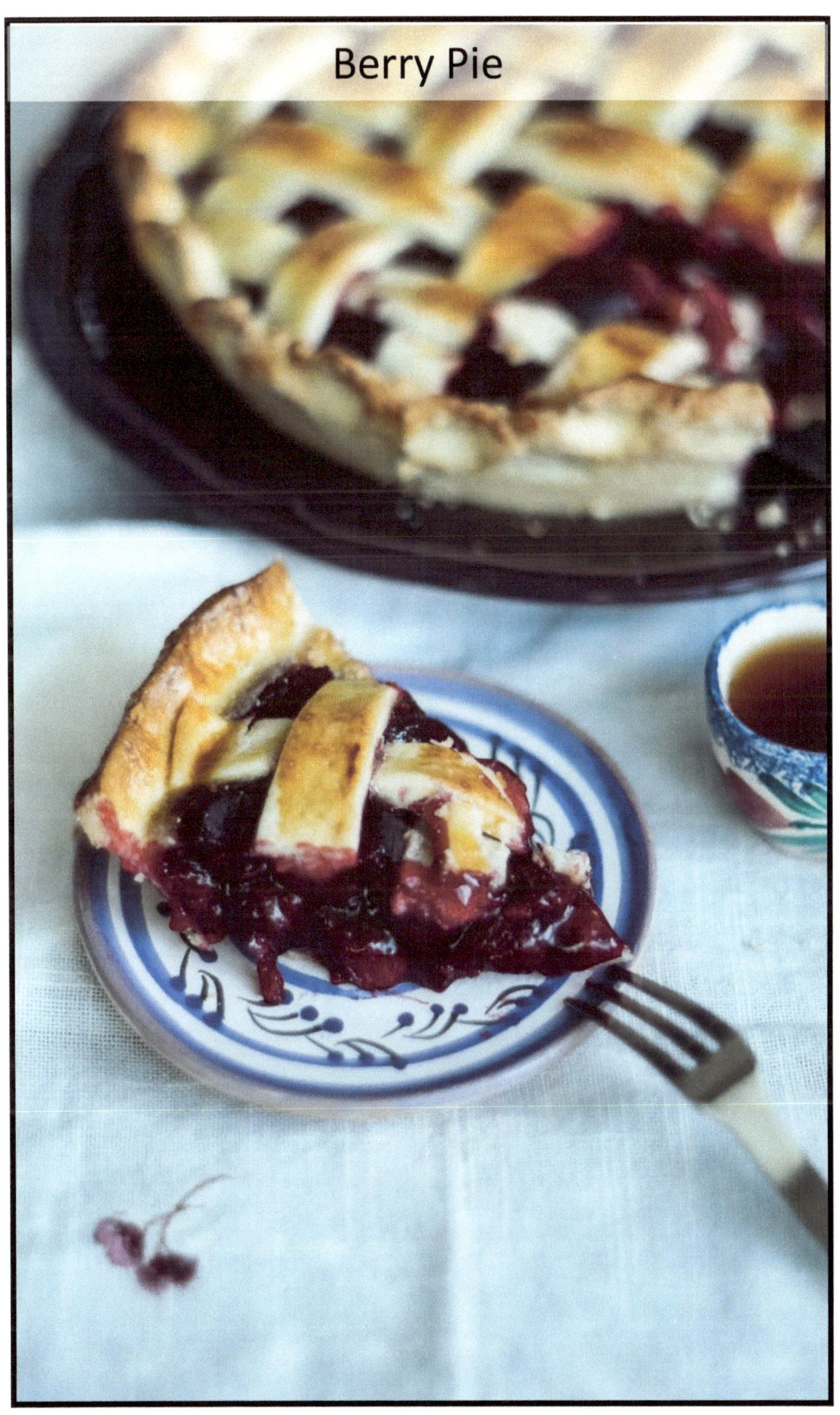

Braided Bread

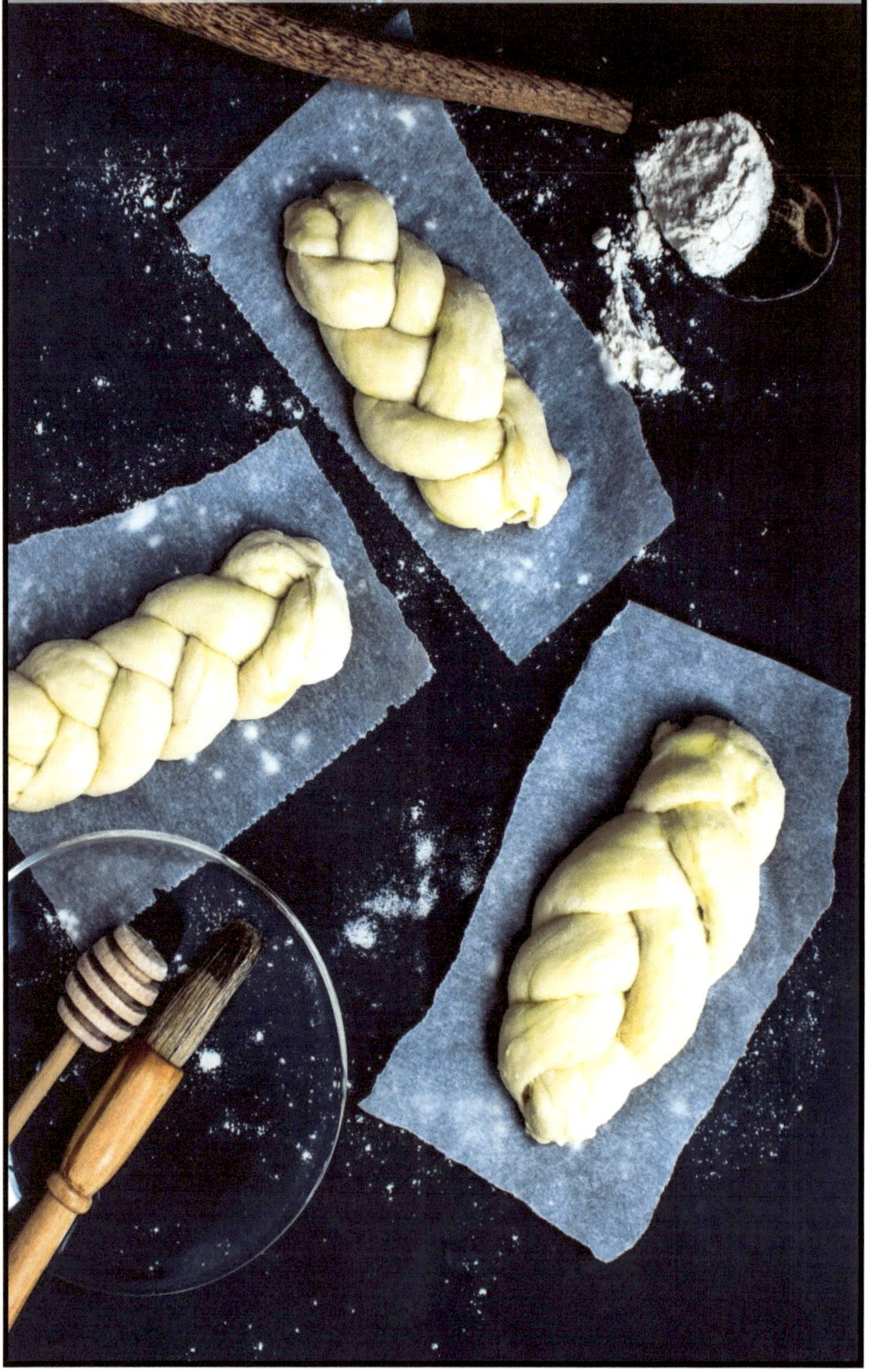

Mixing By Hand

Making Lattice Pie Top

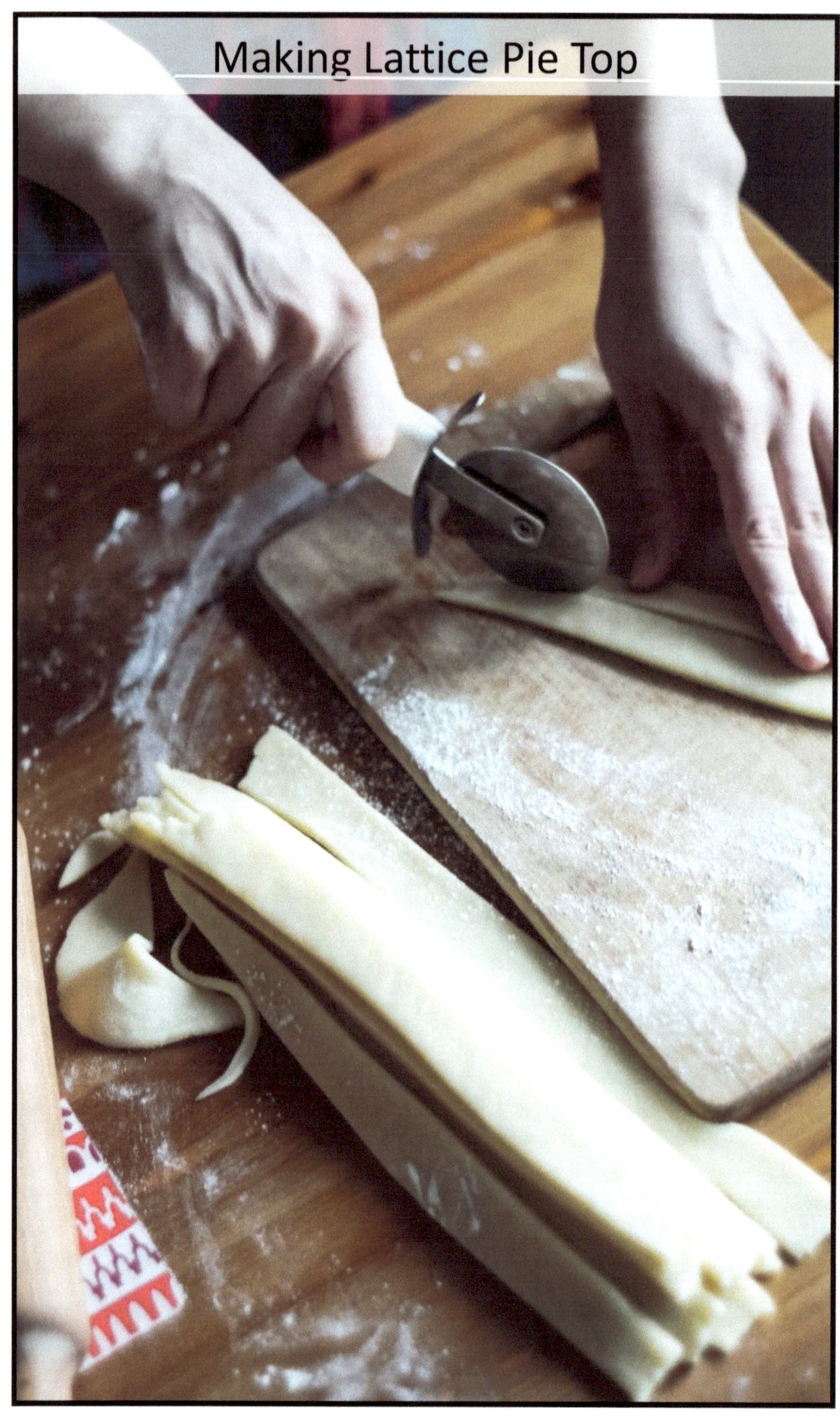

Cutting Biscuits

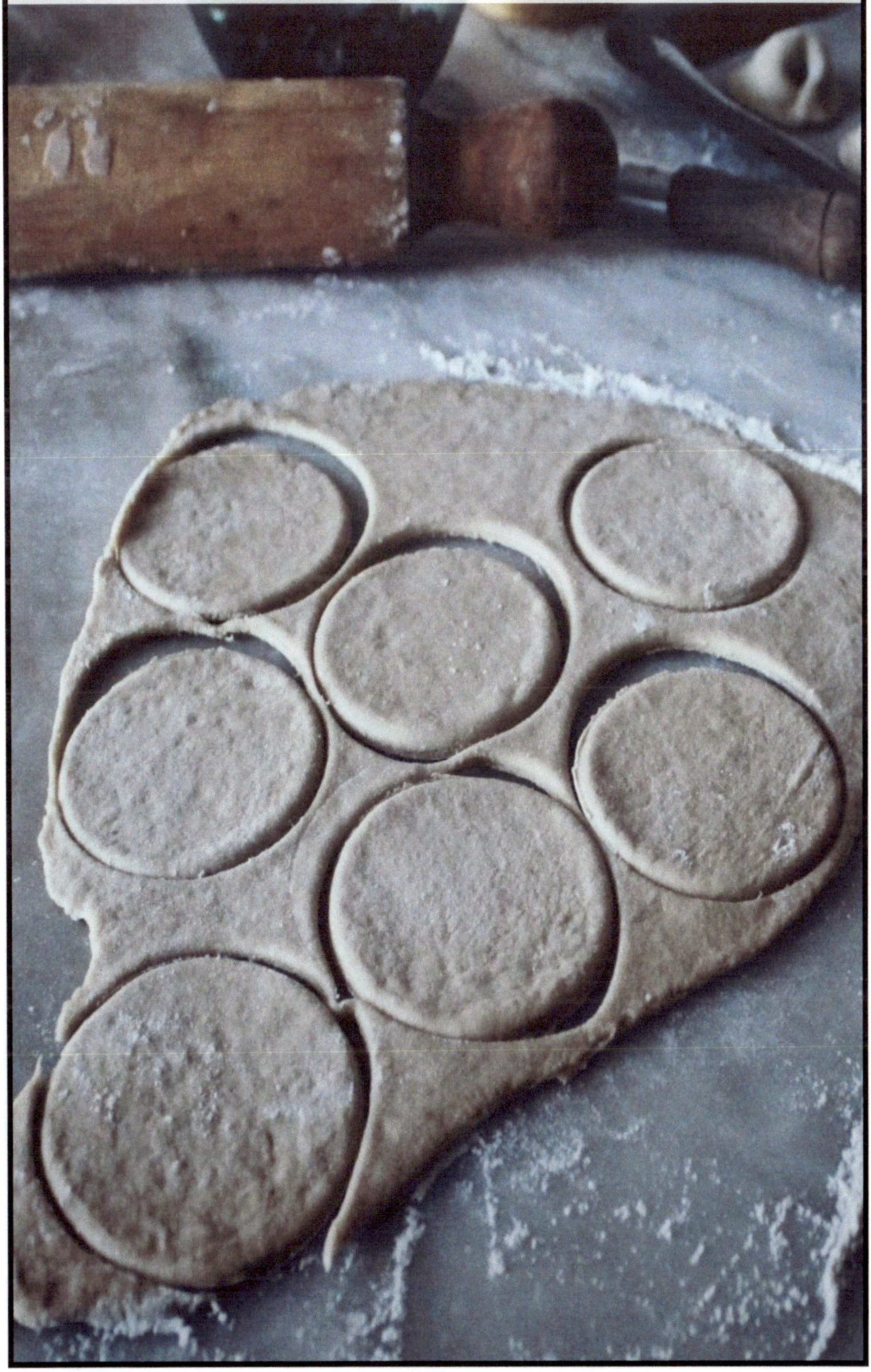

Brownies

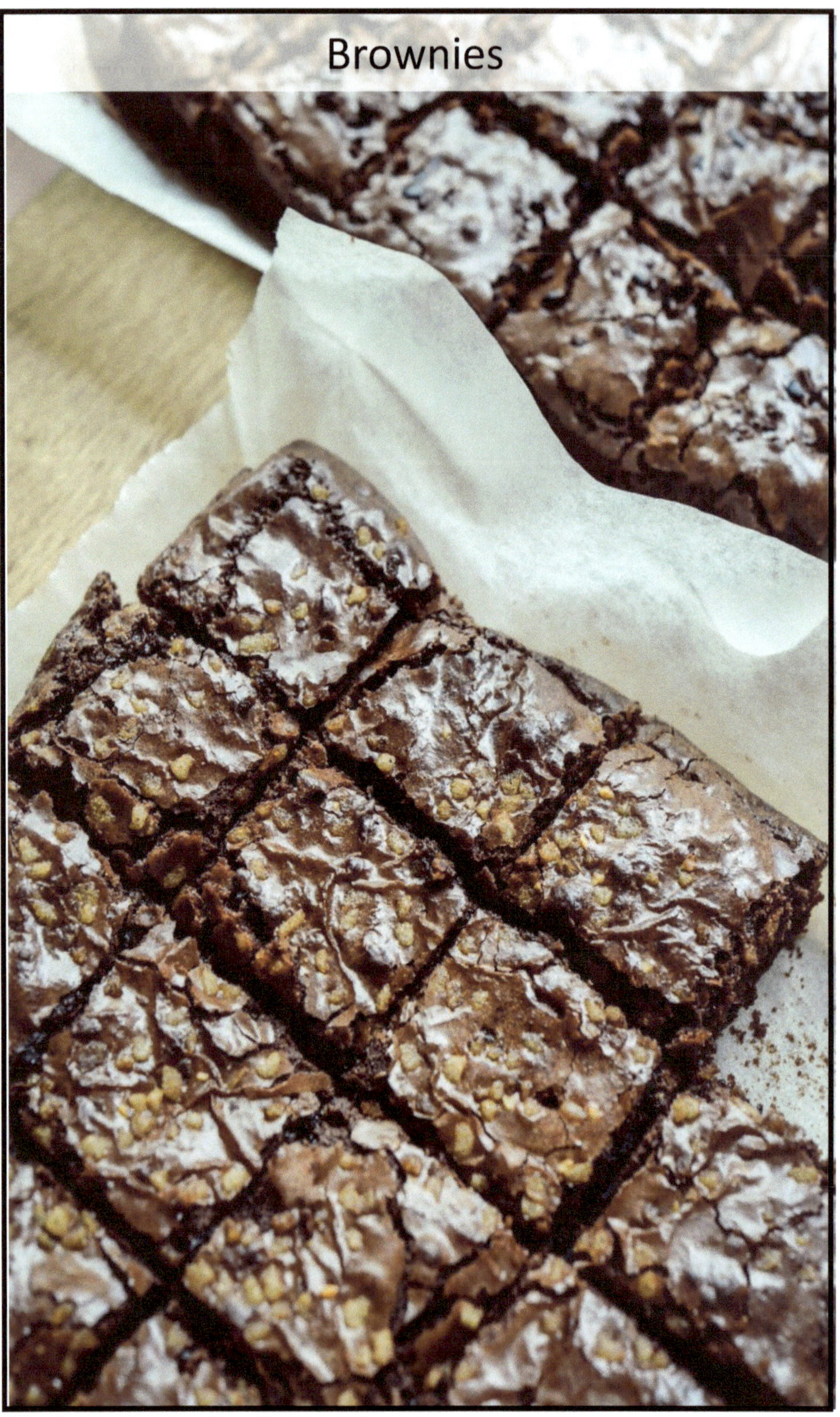

Chocolate Cake

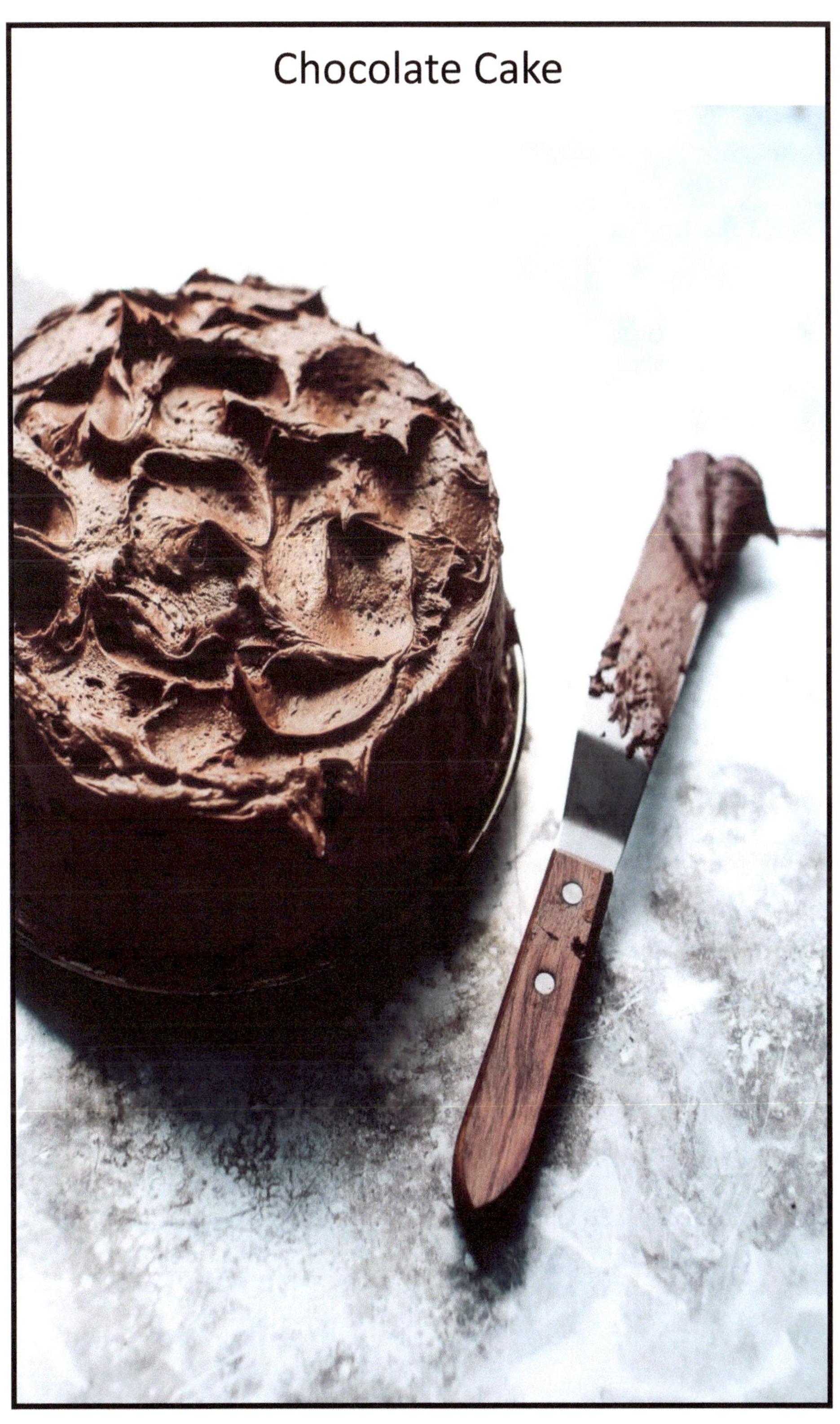

Banana Bread

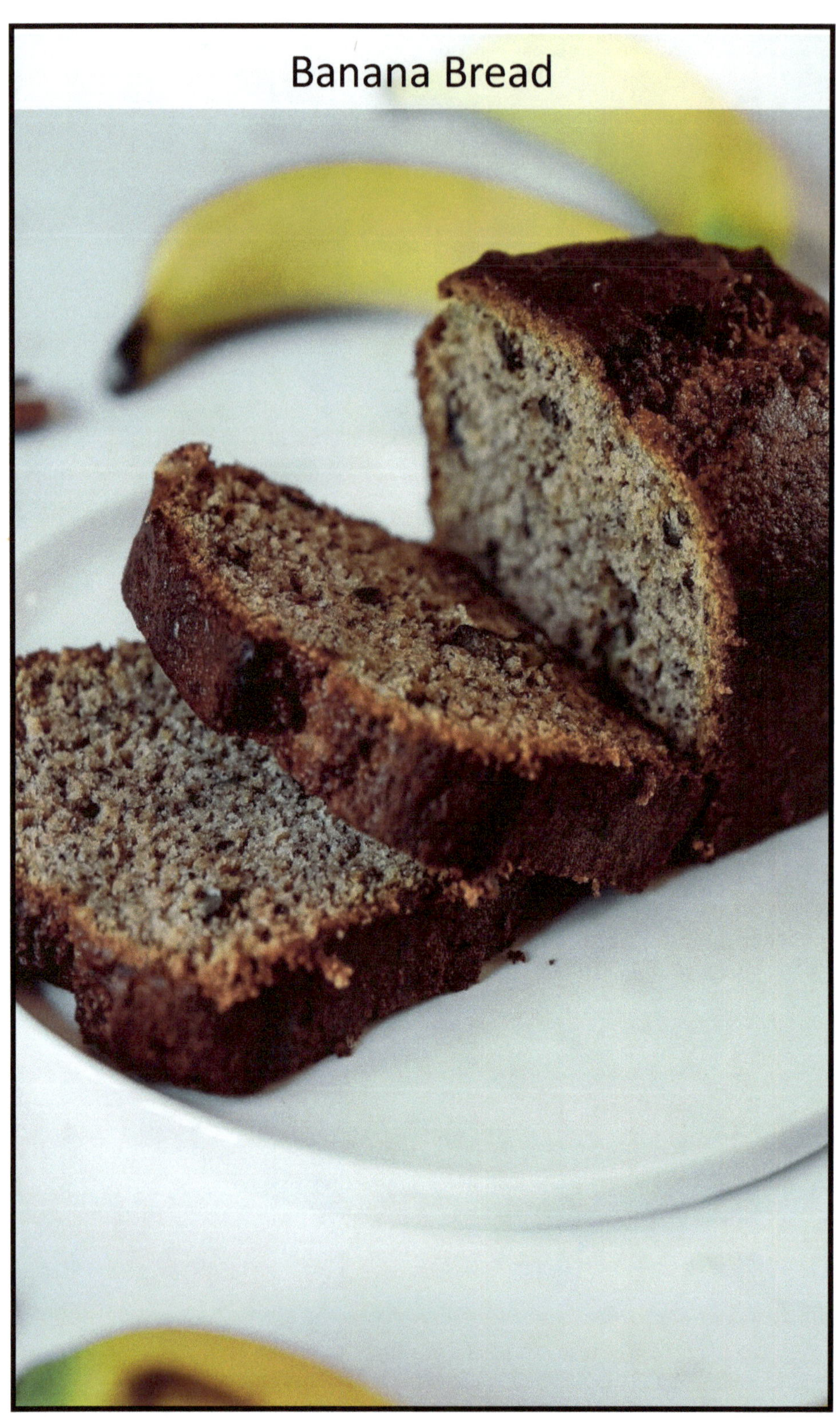

Birthday Cake

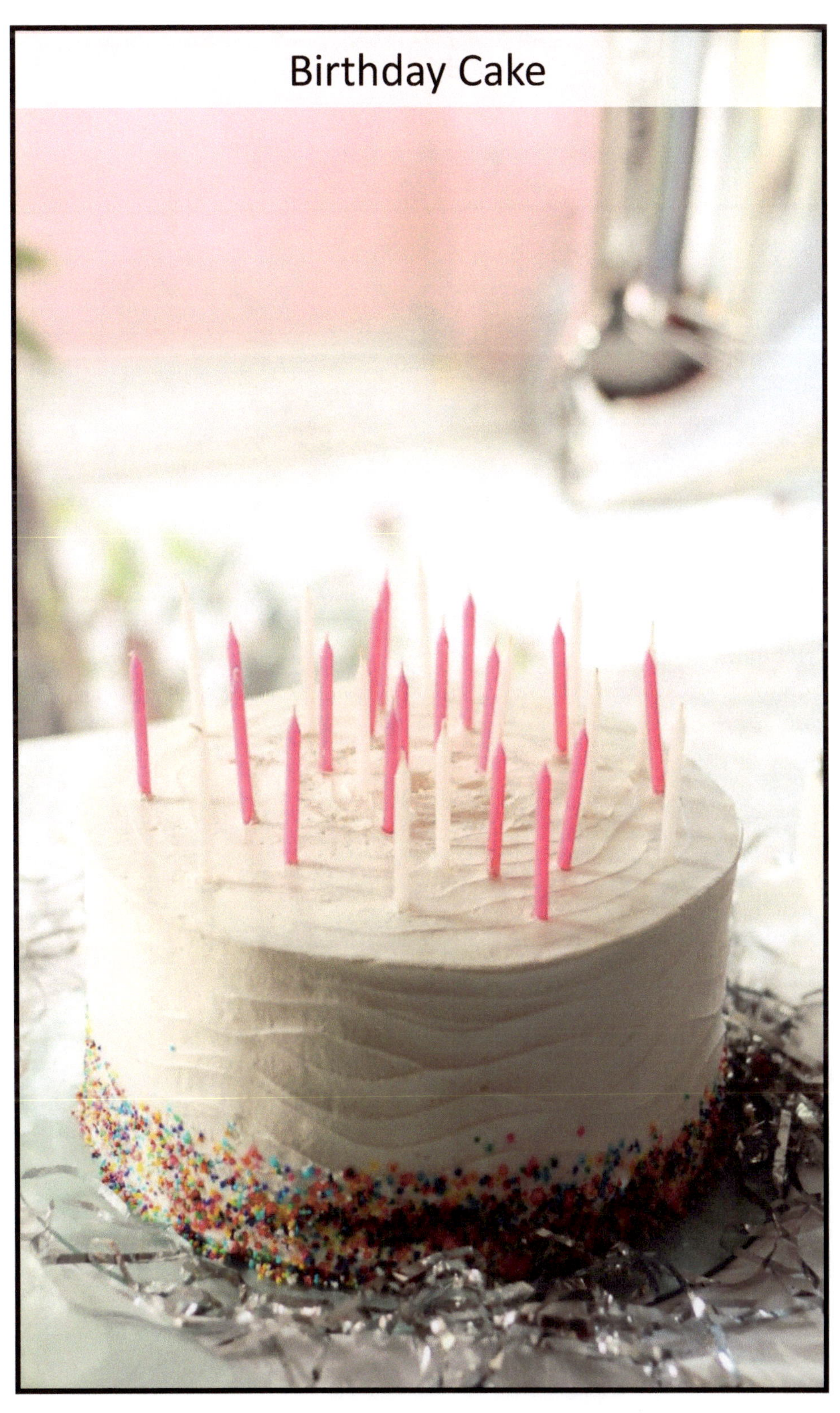

Snickerdoodles

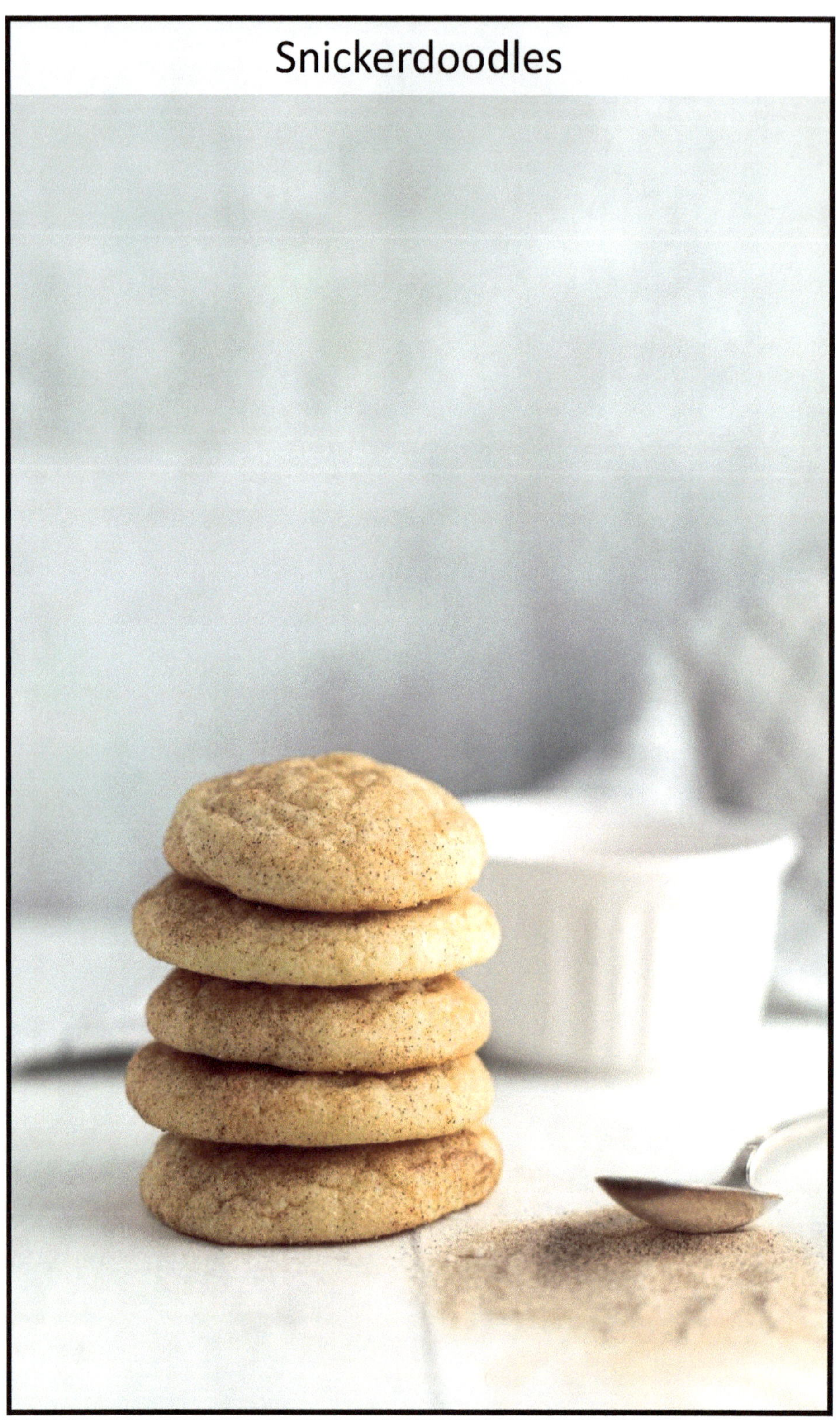

Cheesecake

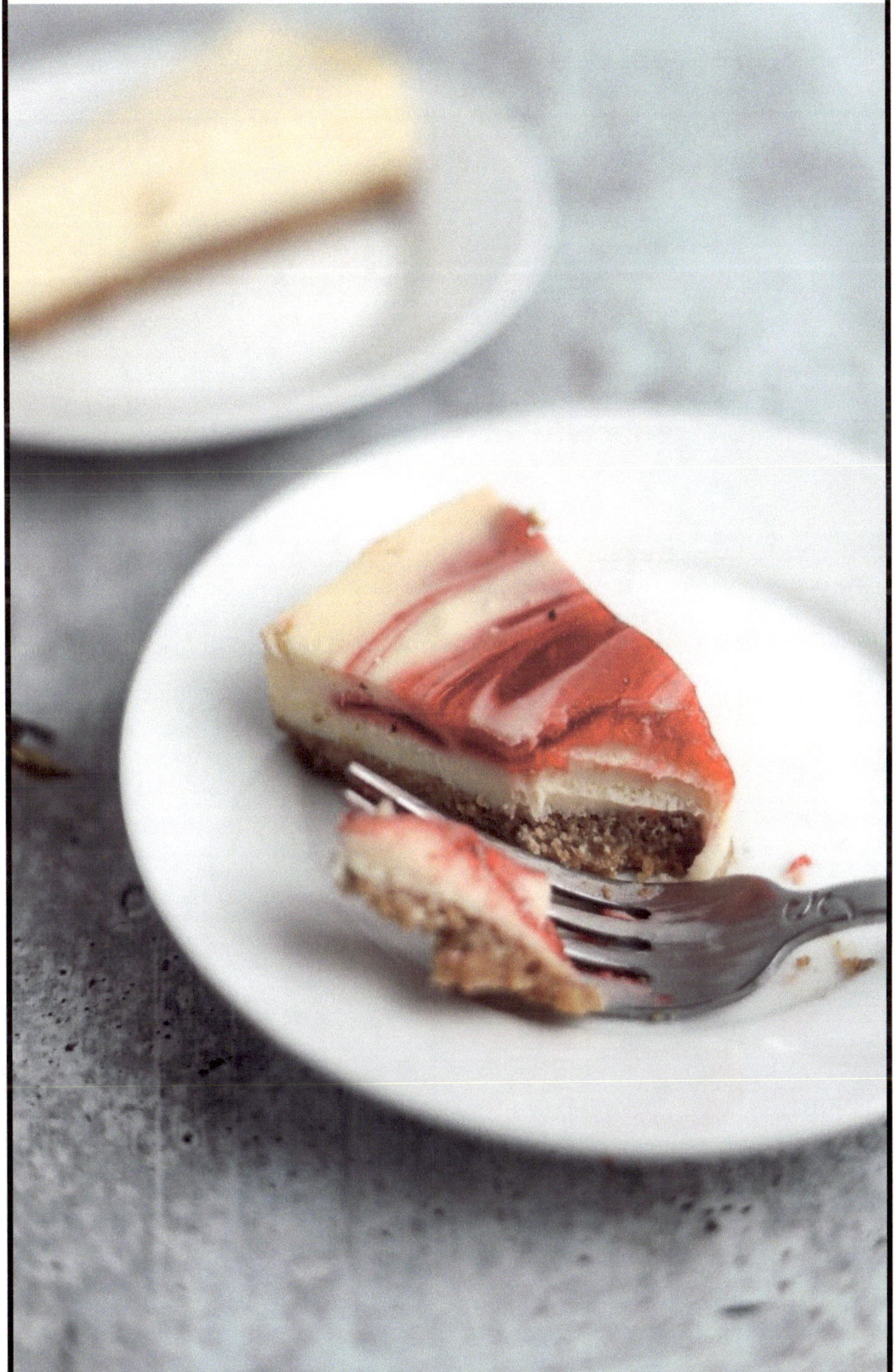

Iced Cookies With Sprinkles

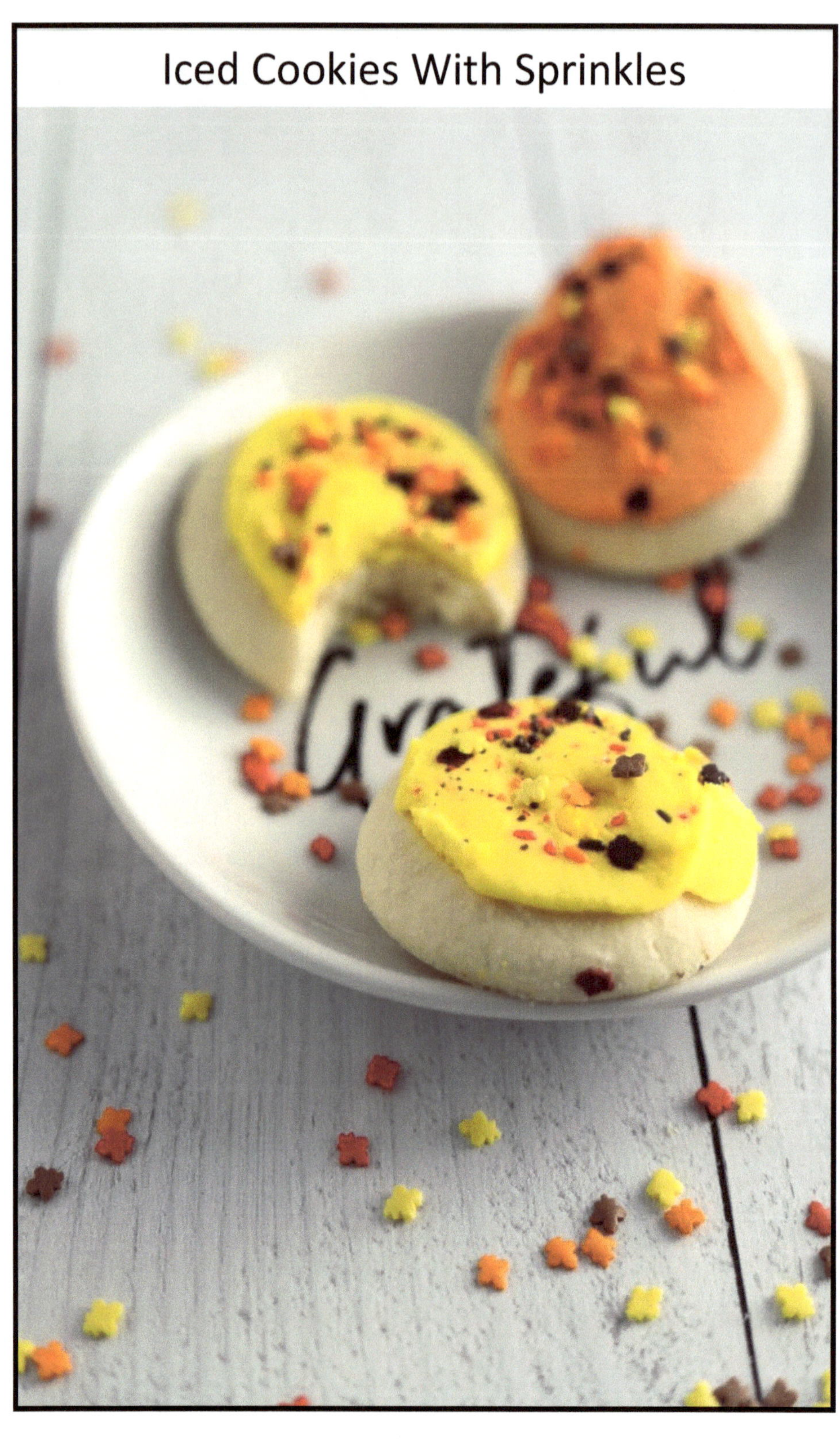

9 798652 103804